Dental and Craniofacial Applications of Platelet-Rich Plasma

Dental and Craniofacial Applications of Platelet-Rich Plasma

Robert E. Marx, DDS
Professor of Surgery and Chief
Division of Oral and Maxillofacial Surgery
Miller School of Medicine
University of Miami
Miami, Florida

Arun K. Garg, DMD
Professor of Surgery
Division of Oral and Maxillofacial Surgery
Miller School of Medicine
University of Miami
Miami, Florida

Quintessence Publishing Co, Inc

Chicago, Berlin, Tokyo, London, Paris, Milan, Barcelona, Istanbul, São Paulo, New Delhi, Moscow, Prague, and Warsaw

Library of Congress Cataloging-in-Publication Data

Marx, Robert E.
  Dental and craniofacial applications of platelet-rich plasma / Robert E.
Marx and Arun K. Garg.
       p. ; cm.
  Includes bibliographical references and index.
  ISBN 0-86715-432-2
  1. Mouth--Surgery. 2. Skull--Surgery. 3. Face--Surgery. 4. Regeneration
(Biology) 5. Blood platelets. 6. Blood plasma.
  [DNLM: 1. Oral Surgical Procedures--methods. 2. Blood
Platelets--physiology. 3. Bone Regeneration--physiology. 4.
Plasma--physiology. 5. Reconstructive Surgical Procedures--methods. 6.
Soft tissue regeneration--physiology. WU 600 M392d 2005] I. Garg, Arun K.,
D.M.D. II. Title.
  RK529.M377 2005
  617.5'22--dc22
                                          2004028665

© 2005 Quintessence Publishing Co, Inc

Quintessence Publishing Co, Inc
551 Kimberly Drive
Carol Stream, Illinois 60188
www.quintpub.com

Editor: Lisa C. Bywaters
Production: Susan Robinson
Cover and internal design: Dawn Hartman

Printed in China

This book is dedicated to the two clinical surgeons/researchers who initiated a paradigm shift that allowed the present generation of researchers to promote tissue regeneration and healing rather than merely removing the obstacles to it: Marshall A. Urist and Thomas K. Hunt.

It was Marshall Urist's 1965 discovery of a remarkable protein residing in living and dead bone that could leach out and influence host cells to form new bone that first revealed the very existence of growth factors and their potential to regenerate tissues. Known as *bone morphogenetic protein* (BMP), this discovery and the pioneering work that followed has not only stood the test of time, but spawned the field of tissue engineering, of which platelet-rich plasma is only a small part. His passing in 2002 saddened all who knew this great scientist/surgeon, but his example stimulated us to continue what he started.

It was Thomas Hunt's 1983 discovery of how macrophages control wound healing by elaborating numerous growth factors and by migrating to a wound in response to oxygen gradients as sensed by surface membrane receptors that established the foundation for our current understanding of wound healing. His precise and diligent research was a model of the scientific method. His articles on the mechanisms of wound healing are classic monographs, and his textbook, *Soft and Hard Tissue Repair* (Praeger, 1984), is considered required reading. Like the principles of Marshall Urist, those of Thomas Hunt have stood the test of time and have spawned the field of tissue engineering. Fortunately for all of us, his work and contributions continue to this day.

Table of Contents

Preface

As of this writing, our understanding of the scientific mechanism of growth factors remains in its infancy. Primitively established in 1965 by the discovery of bone morphogenetic protein, the field of growth factor technology made stellar advances for many years despite a total lack of clinical applications. Beginning in 1998, however, the clinical science of growth factors grew exponentially, primarily as a result of studies involving the composite of growth factors known as *platelet-rich plasma* (PRP). Over the next 7 years, a large body of excellent clinical studies was gradually amassed to define PRP as a legitimate tool in wound healing and essentially the first set of autologous human growth factors directly available to clinical surgeons. PRP is a catalyst for success in routine as well as major reconstructive surgeries and is a critical factor in the healing of compromised wounds. However, it is only an adjunct to healing; it cannot replace the basic principles of sterility, blood supply, and the careful handling of tissues.

This book describes the science, technology, and clinical applications of PRP within several disciplines of dentistry and facial surgery. It shows definitive outcomes and scientific proof of its efficacy as well as the proper techniques necessary to obtain PRP's greatest benefits. This book also answers controversies with scientific data and experience to reassure the reader of the safety of all growth factor applications in addition to those involving PRP. It provides practical information for the reader who wishes to learn phlebotomy techniques, as well as a consent form for harvesting autologous blood, both of which are essential to the clinical application of PRP.

We sincerely hope this book will serve as a useful fund of knowledge as well as a reference, both for newcomers to the field of growth factor technology and for experienced clinical surgeons who wish to expand their use of PRP.

We wish to thank Quintessence Publishing for recognizing the value of PRP and the need for a book on its clinical applications. We thank the entire editorial staff for putting up with our compulsiveness and for helping us gather all of the materials and images into a coherent book. We also extend our sincere gratitude to Maria Ruiz, Executive Secretary of the Division of Oral and Maxillofacial Surgery at the University of Miami, who prepared and made multiple revisions to the manuscript.

I

THE SCIENCE OF PLATELET-RICH PLASMA

chapter one

The Biology of Platelets and the Mechanism of Platelet-Rich Plasma

*"Surgeons do not heal tissue;
they merely place it where nature can heal it."*

Historical Perspective

The limitation of surgery is that it neither guarantees nor even promotes healing. At best, surgeons attempt to remove the known obstacles to healing such as infection, instability, foreign bodies, etc. A review of the literature related to wound healing shows that debridement/primary closure was the "hot topic" of the 1950s. Indeed, soft tissue coverage over exposed bone, traumatic wounds, and surgical defects following proper debridement of nonvital tissue and foreign bodies represented a significant advance in wound healing and remains a basic standard of care to this day. In the 1960s, the focal interest in wound healing was on antibiotics. With the emergence of the cephalosporins and the lincomycin/clindamycin type of antibiotics to complement the penicillins and "sulfa" drugs already in use, surgeons could overcome their main obstacle and nemesis to healing: bacteria. In the 1970s, surgeons realized the benefits of wound stability. Lag screws, rigid plates, and fixation devices were found to enhance vascular ingrowth and cellular proliferation by limiting the micromotion that would shear off newly developing capillaries and inhibit the cellular proliferations required in healing. In the 1980s, the three seminal works by Knighton,[1,2] Hunt,[3] and Marx et al[4,5] identified the pivotal role that oxygen plays in all wound healing. Recognizing that growth factors promote healing, these studies were the first to identify that the macrophage response to oxygen gradients was one of secreting wound-regulating growth factors.[3] This finding marked a paradigm shift by focusing attention on actively promoting healing rather than just removing the obstacles to it. From these basic scientific findings, free vascular transfers,[6] pedicled flaps,[7] and hyperbaric oxygen[8] grew to become standards of care today. Beginning in the 1990s and continuing through the time of this writing (and likely for decades to come), growth factors have emerged as the "Holy Grail" in wound-healing. First introduced clinically by Knighton's platelet-derived wound healing factor (PDWHF)[9] and then through topical recombinant human platelet-derived growth factor bb (PDGFbb) (Regranex, Ortho McNeal) and today's platelet-rich plasma (PRP), platelets have been found to be the pivotal cells that initiate all human wound healing.

The Platelet

Platelets arise from cytoplasmic fragmentation of the megakaryocyte in bone marrow. Like red blood cells, platelets enter the circulation as anuclear cells and therefore have a limited life span. Whereas the red blood cell lives for about 120 days, the platelet lives for only about 7 to 10 days. Although neither of these cells has a nucleus, both are extremely active metabolically. The platelet, in particular, actively synthesizes growth factors throughout its life span and actively secretes them in response to clotting.

A platelet is about 2 μm at its largest diameter, a red blood cell about 8 μm, and a lymphocyte about 12 to 14 μm. The platelet has numerous pseudopodial extensions, invaginations of its cell membrane, and internal vesicles (storage granules). Its morphology is often likened to a natural sea sponge (Fig 1-1) or to Swiss cheese. The vesicles are composed of three types of granules: lysosomal, dense, and alpha. The lysosomal granules seem to function as storage for digestive enzymes. The dense granules mainly store and secrete adenosine diphosphate (ADP), which is a potent recruiter and activator of other platelets. The alpha granules are the storage granules of the growth factors; they contain pre-packaged growth factors in an incomplete and therefore bio-inactive form (Fig 1-2). The growth factors proven to be contained in these granules are the three isomeres of platelet-derived growth factor (PDGFaa, PDGFbb, and PDGFab), the two isomeres of transforming growth factor beta (TGFβ1 and TGFβ2), vascular endothelial growth factor (VEGF), and epithelial growth factor (EGF). The alpha granules are also rich in the cell adhesion molecule vitronectin, which is required for osteoconduction and osseointegration. Platelets do not contain insulin-like growth factors (ILG$_1$ or ILG$_2$) or bone morphogenetic protein (BMP).

The circulating platelet participates in natural wound healing based on its numbers in circulating blood. It further participates in enhanced wound healing by virtue of its increased concentration in PRP. In both situations its secretion of growth factors is activated by the clotting process. The activation of the clotting process is associated with a structural change in the platelet membrane system and results in the active secretion of the growth factors from the alpha granules.

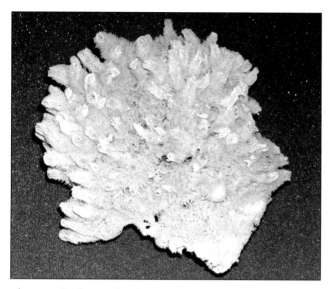

Fig 1-1 The internal cell membrane network, surface invaginations, and vesicles of a platelet give it an appearance similar to that of a sea sponge.

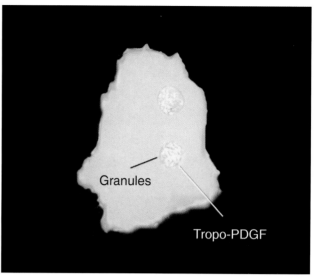

Fig 1-2 The alpha granules in platelets contain incomplete protein and bio-inactive growth factors.

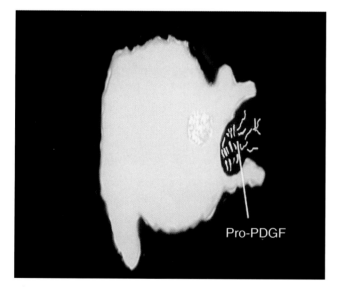

Fig 1-3 The clotting process induces migration of the alpha granules to the cell surface, where the membrane of the alpha granules fuses to the platelet surface membrane.

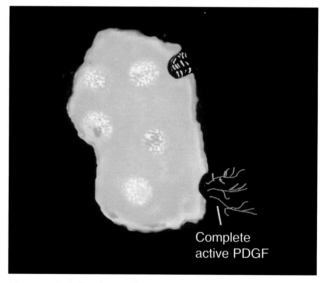

Fig 1-4 The platelet surface membrane adds carbohydrate side chains and histones to the growth factors to make them bioactive.

The alpha granules migrate to the platelet surface membrane and fuse to it (Fig 1-3). The incomplete growth factor proteins (note that all growth factors are proteins) are acted upon by the cell membrane. Histone and carbohydrate side chains are added to these proteins. Then, and only then, are the growth factors biologically active (Fig 1-4).

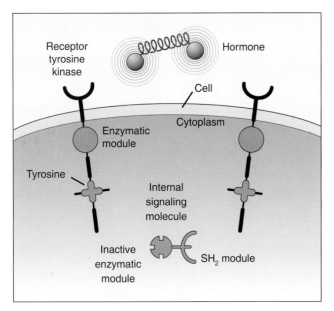

Fig 1-5 The growth factors bind to membrane receptor sites on a target cell. These receptors have both external and intracytoplasmic internal components and are thus termed *transmembrane receptors*.

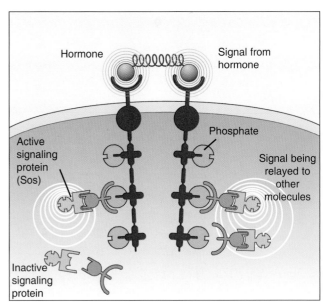

Fig 1-6 Activation of the external receptor site causes a high-energy phosphate bond activation of an intracytoplasmic transducer protein.

The Mechanism of PRP Related to Growth Factors

The growth factors secreted by the platelets (ie, PDGFaa, PDGFbb, and PDGFab) usually have two active sites and are therefore called *dimers*. They attach only to cells that have receptors to accommodate them. These receptors are on the surface membrane of the target cell. The growth factor never enters the target cell; instead, it activates the membrane receptor, which has an intracytoplasmic portion and therefore is often termed a *transmembrane receptor* (Fig 1-5). Two adjacent transmembrane receptors are then brought within a critical distance of each other to activate dormant intracytoplasmic signal transducer proteins (Fig 1-6). A signal transducer protein then detaches from the transmembrane receptor and floats in the cytoplasm toward the nucleus (Figs 1-7 to 1-9). In the nucleus, the transducer protein unlocks a specific gene sequence for a regulated cellular function, such as mitosis, collagen synthesis, osteoid production, etc. The significance of this process is that it explains why an exogenous application of growth factors, even in the highest concentration possible, cannot produce a sustained overreaction such as a hyperplasia, a benign tumor, or a malignant tumor. Growth factors are not mutagenic; they are natural proteins acting through normal gene regulation and normal wound-healing feedback control mechanisms.[10]

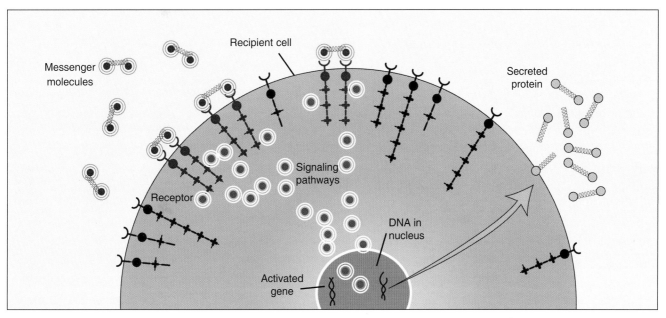

Fig 1-7 The activated signal transducer protein detaches from the transmembrane receptor, floats in the cytoplasm, and enters the nucleus to induce expression of a normal gene.

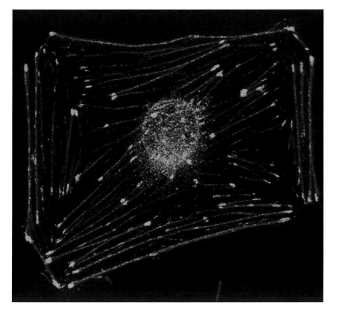

Fig 1-8 Isolated target cell before growth factor binding to membrane receptors. (Courtesy of Lorene Langeberg, Vollum Institute.)

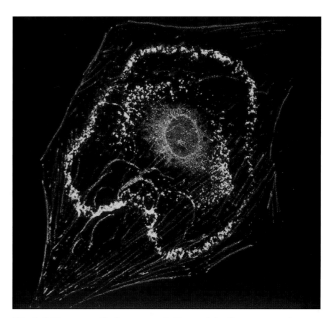

Fig 1-9 Target cell after growth factor binding to membrane receptors shows immunofluorescent signal transducer proteins floating to the nucleus and an expansion of the nuclear membrane. (Courtesy of Lorene Langeberg, Vollum Institute.)

Characterization of the Growth Factors Contained in Platelets

Platelet-derived growth factors

The three PDGFs (PDGFaa, PDGFbb, and PDGFab) are isomeres of one protein measuring approximately 25,000 d each. Each isomere has a slightly different action, and many of these actions overlap. The PDGFs are the most universal growth factors in wound healing. Essentially mitogens, they induce replication in cells that possess membrane receptors specific to them. They stimulate mesenchymal stem cells to replicate, osteoblasts to replicate and produce osteoid, endothelial cells to replicate and secrete basal lamina for new blood vessels, and fibroblasts to replicate and produce collagen.

Transforming growth factors

TGFβ1 and TGFβ2 are just two growth factors in the so-called super family of TGFβs, which contains at least 47 known growth factors. (The BMPs are also within this super family.) TGFβ1 and TGFβ2 are protein growth factors that, like the PDGFs, stimulate cell replication, but they also stimulate matrix production and guide differentiation toward cartilage or bone. Therefore, the TGFβs are also morphogens.

Vascular endothelial growth factor

VEGF is another protein growth factor. Its effects are limited to endothelial cells, the stimulation of basal lamina synthesis, and the recruitment of pericytes to support new blood vessel development.

Epithelial growth factor

EGF also is a protein growth factor. Its effects are limited to the basal cells of skin and mucous membrane. It induces replication, migration over a biologic surface, and stimulation of these cells to lay down the specific components of the basement membrane.

What is PRP?

PRP is an otherwise normal autogenous blood clot that contains a highly concentrated number of platelets. Because it is the patient's own blood, it is free of transmissible diseases and cannot cause hypersensitivity reactions. The minimum platelet count required for a blood clot to qualify as PRP may be arguable, but a concentration of about 1 million platelets/μL, or about 4 to 7 times the usual baseline platelet

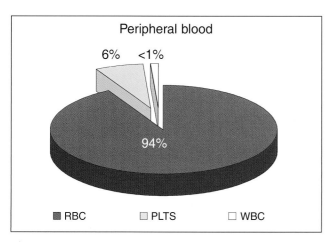

Fig 1-10 Cell ratios in a normal blood clot. (RBC, red blood cells; PLTS, platelets; WBC, white blood cells.)

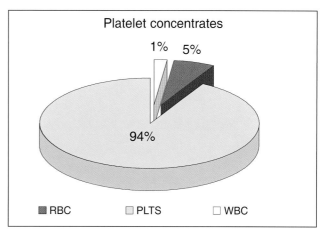

Fig 1-11 Cell ratios in a PRP blood clot. (RBC, red blood cells; PLTS, platelets; WBC, white blood cells.)

count (ie, 200,000 platelets/μL) has been shown to provide clinical benefits.[11] A normal blood clot such as that found in a wound resulting from an implant drill site, a tooth socket, or a bone graft contains 94% red blood cells, 6% platelets, and somewhat less than 1% white blood cells (Fig 1-10). In contrast, a PRP blood clot contains 94% platelets, only 5% red blood cells, and 1% white blood cells (Fig 1-11). This alteration of the cellular ratios in the wound blood clot, whereby cells that do not stimulate healing (red blood cells) are replaced by cells that stimulate all phases of healing (platelets), explains its ability to enhance healing. It also underscores the simple strategy and benefit of PRP, which is to increase the growth factor actions on healing and bone regeneration by increasing the numbers of platelets.

Mechanisms of Platelets and PRP in Bone Regeneration

The alpha granules contained in platelets, whether in a normal blood clot or in a PRP clot, begin degranulating within 10 minutes of clot development and secrete over 90% of their pre-packaged growth factors within 1 hour. The growth factors immediately bind to the transmembrane receptors of osteoprogenitor cells, endothelial cells, and mesenchymal stem cells. The fibrin and fibronectin contained within the acellular portion of the clot and the vitronectin arising from the platelet alpha granules envelop the graft in an initial matrix. The three isomeres of PDGF act as mitogens for osteoblast, endothelial cell, and mesenchymal stem cell proliferation. The two TGFβ isomeres accomplish a similar mitogenesis and angiogenesis but also promote osteoblastic differentiation of the mesenchymal stem cells. The VEGF promotes specific capillary ingrowth. The EGF is likely to be nonfunctional due to the absence of epithelial cells (Fig 1-12).

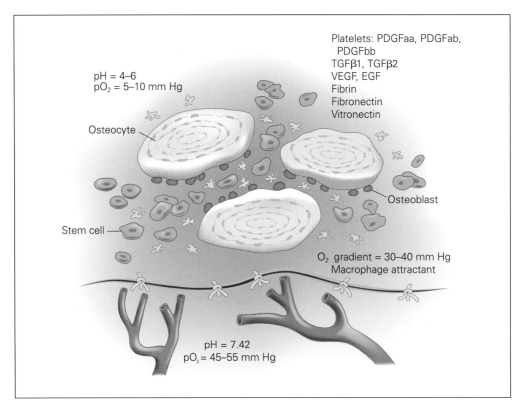

pH = 4–6
pO$_2$ = 5–10 mm Hg

Platelets: PDGFaa, PDGFab,
    PDGFbb
TGFβ1, TGFβ2
VEGF, EGF
Fibrin
Fibronectin
Vitronectin

Osteocyte

Osteoblast

Stem cell

O$_2$ gradient = 30–40 mm Hg
Macrophage attractant

pH = 7.42
pO$_2$ = 45–55 mm Hg

Fig 1-12 The biochemical environment of an autogenous bone graft.

Because of its increased concentration of platelets, the PRP thus initiates a greater and faster initial cellular response in the bone graft than the normal blood clot. Identifiable osteoprogenitor cell mitosis and capillary buds can be seen as early as 3 days after graft placement (Fig 1-13). By 17 to 21 days, the capillary penetration of the graft is complete and the osteoprogenitor cells have vastly increased in number (Fig 1-14). Thus, the first phase of bone graft healing occurs during the first 3 weeks and is characterized by capillary ingrowth and rapid cellular metabolism, proliferation, and activity. It is during this phase that the graft is most vulnerable to infection and instability, either of which can prevent, or lyse, the delicate cells and cellular functions occurring during this time. The clinician who understands this will take measures to ensure that the tissue is infection- and contamination-free and will provide absolute graft stability during this time period.

Although the platelets are exhausted within 7 to 10 days, their effect on graft development has been established. The platelets have by this time dictated the rate and degree of bone regeneration. The circulating macrophage and the blood monocyte, which becomes a wound macrophage, are attracted to the wound environment mainly by its hypoxic nature and to a lesser degree by lactate and acidity. Macrophages possess membrane receptors that sense areas of low oxygen concentration. The inherent hypoxia of an early bone graft holds a strong attraction for the macrophage, which arrives at the wound and secretes additional growth factors to regulate and continue the bone regeneration. Not to be overlooked is

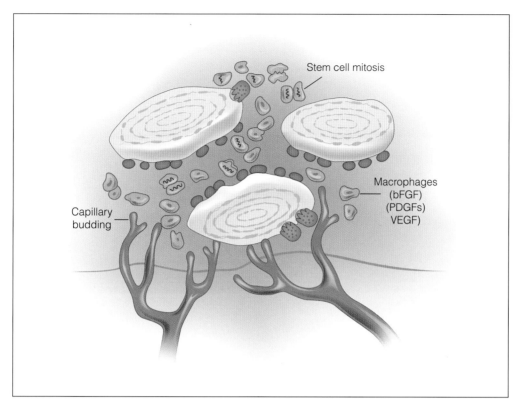

Fig 1-13 As early as 3 days after graft placement, significant cell divisions and penetration of capillary buds into the graft can be seen.

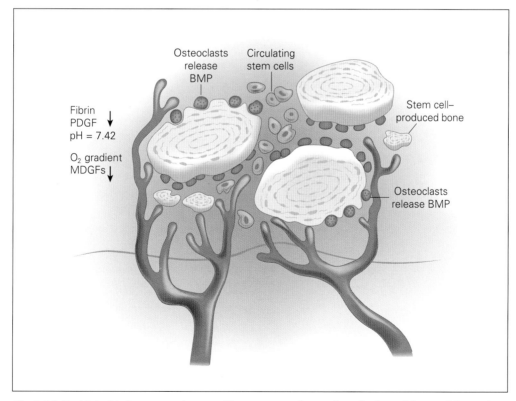

Fig 1-14 By 17 to 21 days, complete capillary penetration and profusion of the graft has taken place, and osteoid production has been initiated.

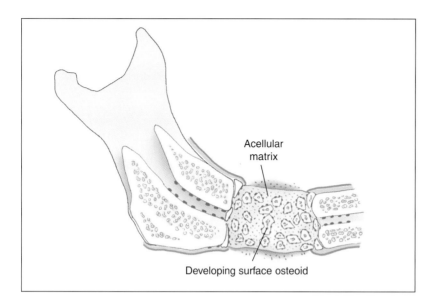

Fig 1-15a Acellular matrix along with surface osteoid developing on the endosteal surfaces of the transplanted bone and the resection edges of the host bone in a 3-week autogenous bone graft.

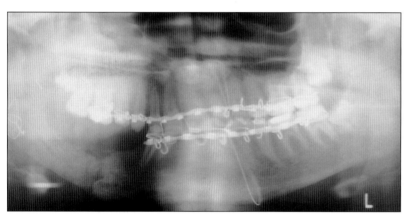

Fig 1-15b Corresponding radiograph shows a not-yet-mineralized graft with a "cloudy" appearance indicative of a graft that is not yet consolidated. The radiolucent line between the graft and host bone is the result of a dying-back resorption of the host bone from periosteal reflection.

the meshed clot itself, which contains fibrin, fibronectin, and vitronectin. These cell adhesion molecules act as a surface matrix for the vascular ingrowth, cell proliferation, and cell migration occurring during this phase. This matrix will also act as the initial scaffold for osteoid production that will signal the transition to the next stage.

Between 3 and 6 weeks, the osteoprogenitor cells have proliferated and differentiated sufficiently to produce osteoid (Figs 1-15a and 1-15b). Their production of osteoid consolidates the graft and forms a union to the adjacent native bone (Figs 1-16a and 1-16b); this is often described as the second phase of bone regeneration. During this time the completed capillary ingrowth matures by developing adventitial supporting cells around the vessels, making them much more capable of withstanding instability and mild function. The oxygen that these vessels supply to the graft reverses the hypoxia and thus downregulates the macrophage so that the wound does not "overheal" into a hyperplasia. Beginning at the 6th week, the osteoid undergoes an obligatory resorption-remodeling cycle (Fig 1-17). The weak and elastic osteoid is resorbed by osteoclasts, which release BMPs, ILG_1, and ILG_2, and these in turn induce adjacent osteoblasts and mesenchymal stem cells to differentiate and produce a more mature replacement bone (Fig 1-18) that contains

Fig 1-16a By fusing graft particles together and to the host bone, the graft has produced sufficient osteoid to consolidate by 6 weeks.

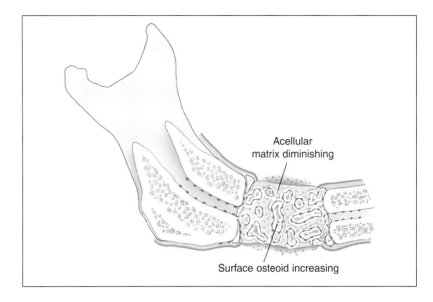

Fig 1-16b Corresponding radiograph shows condensation of the cloudy graft appearance, indicative of osteoid production and graft organization. The radiolucent line between the graft and host bone has nearly disappeared as a result of osteoconduction between the graft and host bone edge.

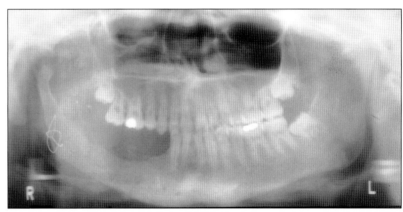

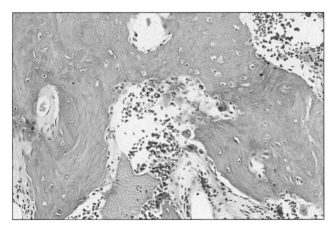

Fig 1-17 At about 6 weeks, the graft begins a major resorption-remodeling cycle in which osteoclasts resorb the disorganized immature bone and release BMP and ILG, thus inducing formation of new bone that will mature during function.

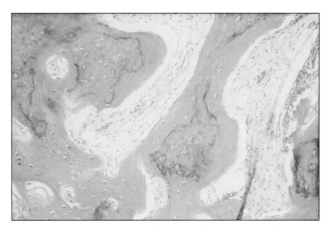

Fig 1-18 Transitional stage between immature and mature bone. The immature bone is more cellular, has larger cells, and is random compared to the more mature replacement bone.

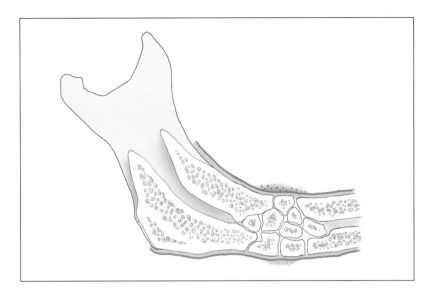

Fig 1-19a After 6 weeks, the graft will be consolidated and fused to the host bone. It then enters the lifelong resorption-remodeling cycle of the remainder of the skeleton.

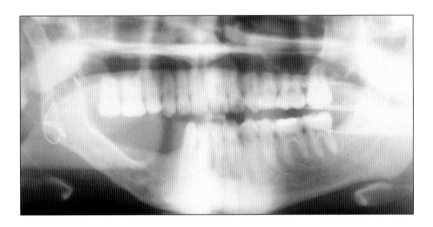

Fig 1-19b Radiographically, bone maturation is characterized by the development of a normal trabecular pattern and an increased density. Here, an inferior border outline, an external oblique ridge, and a coronoid process attest to the remodeling of bone under function.

lamellar architecture and Haversian systems not present in osteoid. This third phase of bone regeneration continues throughout the lifetime of the graft as it settles into the normal resorption-remodeling turnover rate of the rest of the skeleton (about 0.7% per day). This is seen clinically and radiographically by the formation of mineralized dense bone (Figs 1-19a and 1-19b).

Thus, platelets and PRP act in the early biochemical first phase of a three-phase bone-regeneration sequence, when the pivotal role of setting the rate and amount of bone regeneration takes place.

Clinical Effects of PRP on Bone Regeneration

The seminal study validating the concentration of platelets and their stimulation of bone graft healing appeared in *Oral Surgery, Oral Medicine, Oral Pathology, Oral Radiology, and Endodontics* in 1998[11] and documented that PRP is a concentration

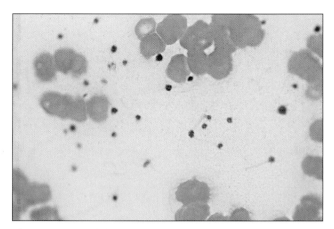

Fig 1-20a A peripheral blood smear shows a minimal number of platelets interspersed with red blood cells.

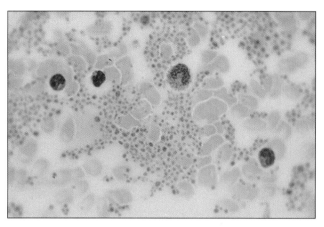

Fig 1-20b A PRP smear developed from the same blood used in Fig 1-20a shows a tremendously increased number of platelets interspersed with red blood cells, as well as a few white blood cells.

Fig 1-21 Immunoperoxidase stain of an autogenous graft showing that the brown-staining osteoprogenitor cells have membrane receptors to TGFβ1. Note that osteoblasts remain as osteoprogenitor cells whereas mature osteocytes do not. Also, the highest concentration of osteoprogenitor cells is seen as the perivascular cells around a venule identifying the pericyte as a bone regenerative cell.

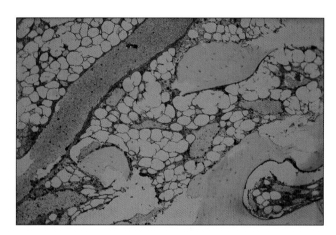

of platelets 4 to 7 times above baseline peripheral blood platelet levels (Figs 1-20a and 1-20b).

The study further demonstrated that bone graft cells do indeed possess membrane receptors for nearly all of the growth factors contained within platelets (Fig 1-21). In addition, radiographs and computerized tomography (CT) scans showed an increase in bone mineral density in PRP-supported grafts that ranged from 1.6 to 2.2 times that of non-PRP-supported grafts (Figs 1-22a and 1-22b; Table 1-1). This increase indicated a clinically more rapid formation and earlier maturation of the bone grafts that were stimulated by the PRP. Histomorphometry showed that while autogenous bone grafts without PRP enhancement produced a trabecular bone value of 55% ± 8% (Fig 1-23) (compared to a native mandible value of 38% ± 6% [Fig 1-24]), the PRP-enhanced grafts produced a value of 74% ± 11% (Fig 1-25). This measure indicated an increased density of bone produced by the PRP as well as an advanced rate of maturity (Table 1-2).

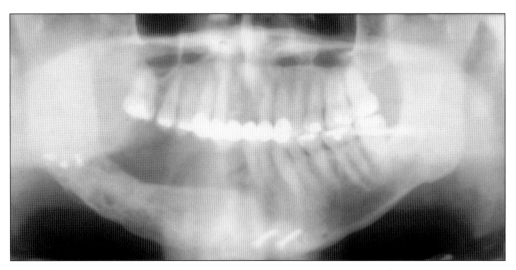

Fig 1-22a Panoramic radiograph of a hemimandibular autogenous bone graft at 4 months showing excellent bone formation and continuity interrupted by areas of immaturity.

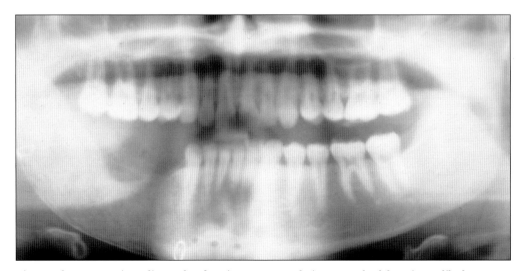

Fig 1-22b Panoramic radiograph of a size-, age-, and time-matched hemimandibular autogenous bone graft enhanced with PRP showing greater bone density indicative of advanced maturity.

Table 1-1	Graft Maturity Index		
	2 mos	4 mos	6 mos
Grafts without PRP (44)	0.92	0.88	1.06
Grafts with PRP (44)	2.16	1.88	1.62
	(P = .001)	(P = .001)	(P = .001)

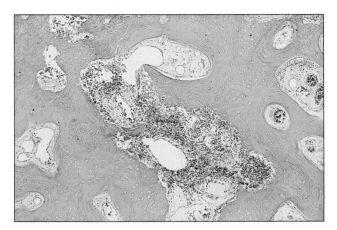

Fig 1-23 Histomorphometry of an autogenous bone graft without PRP at 4 months shows that the graft has a 60% trabecular bone density, consists mostly of immature bone, and is undergoing active resorption-remodeling.

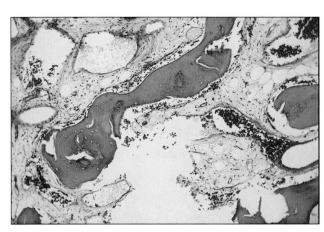

Fig 1-24 Histomorphometry of a native posterior mandible serves as a baseline. It contains 38% trabecular bone area consisting of mature bone within a fibrovascular stroma.

Fig 1-25 Histomorphometry of an autogenous bone graft enhanced with PRP at 4 months shows that the graft has an 80% bone density, consists almost entirely of mature bone with lamellar architecture, and features mature Haversian systems with limited bone remodeling.

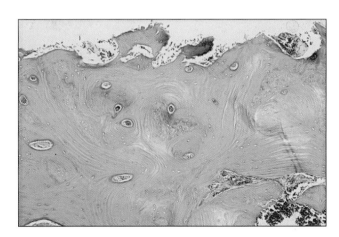

Table 1-2	Histomorphometry of Autogenous Bone Grafts at 6 Months	
Type of bone	Trabecular bone area	
Native mandible (1)	38.9% ± 6%	
Grafts without PRP (44)	55.0% ± 8%	(P = .005)
Grafts with PRP (44)	74.0% ± 11%	(P = .005)

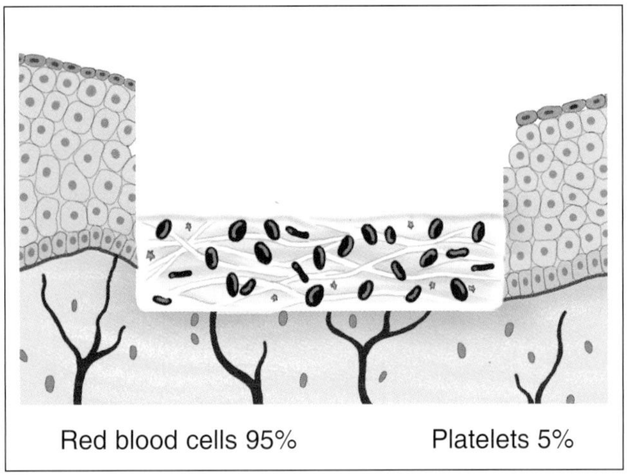

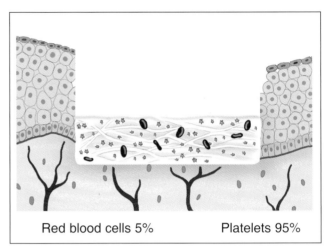

Fig 1-26a A split-thickness skin graft without PRP forms a surface clot containing 5% platelets and 95% red blood cells within a fibrin network.

Fig 1-26b A split-thickness skin graft enhanced with PRP forms a surface clot containing 95% platelets and 5% red blood cells within a fibrin network.

Effects of PRP on Soft Tissue Healing

The effects of PRP on soft tissue healing parallel those in bone regeneration but often seem to be even more dramatic because the enhancement of healing is more readily observable. The best model for demonstrating PRP enhancement of soft tissue healing is a split-thickness skin graft donor site.[12] A randomized prospective study was performed on adjacent skin graft donor site wounds that were a standard size of 4 × 7 cm and a standard depth of 0.42 mm. One wound was treated with only topical bovine thrombin as a hemostatic agent and the other with PRP activated with topical bovine thrombin. The PRP-enhanced site showed a dramatic clinical and histologic difference, displaying the healing enhancement afforded by PRP.

A split-thickness skin graft donor site wound is excavated below the basement membrane level; it therefore heals by capillary budding from its connective tissue base and epithelial migration through the nutritional support from the capillary perfusion, mostly from the skin edges and to a lesser degree from hair follicle epithelium. Once the skin graft is removed, a blood clot forms on the connective tissue base (Fig 1-26a). The platelets within the blood clot degranulate to secrete their seven growth factors, while the fibrin, fibronectin, and vitronectin cell adhesion molecules coat the surface as a matrix for cell migration. The VEGF and the three PDGF isomeres induce a rapid capillary proliferation to produce a nutritional supply within the wound. The TGFβ isomeres stimulate fibroplasia and collagen synthesis at the wound base. Most importantly, however, EGF acts upon the basal cells at the wound edge (basal cells are the stem cells of epithelium) to promote an epithelial proliferation, which will migrate into the nutrient-rich granulation tissue on the surface of the cell adhesion molecules in the clot.

Replacing the normal clot that develops in this soft tissue wound with a PRP clot increases the growth factors available to it (Fig 1-26b). In the study described above,

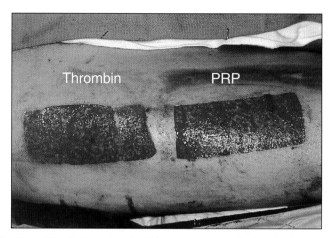

Fig 1-27a Adjacent split-thickness skin graft donor sites at time of harvest. One site has a thrombin-activated normal blood clot, the other a thrombin-activated PRP clot. Note that above the PRP clot is an older skin graft donor site that shows significant scarring, contraction, and pigment alteration.

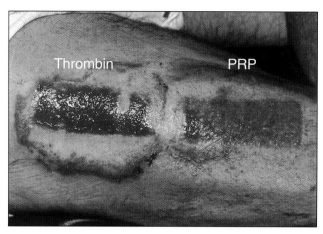

Fig 1-27b The same donor sites at 6 days. The normal clot donor site has a peripheral erythema and exuberant granulation tissue with minimal epithelial ingrowth. The PRP-enhanced donor site has no peripheral erythema and a nearly complete epithelial covering at this early time frame.

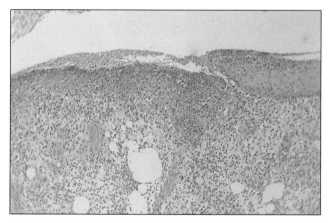

Fig 1-28a Histology from the 6-day split-thickness skin graft donor site not enhanced with PRP shows no epithelial budding and numerous plump immature fibroblasts and macrophages within a granulation tissue base.

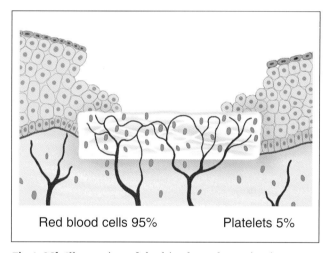

Red blood cells 95%   Platelets 5%

Fig 1-28b Illustration of the histology shown in Fig 1-28a.

a 6-day clinical view of the blood clot site versus the PRP clot site showed a significant acceleration of the healing process in the site with PRP despite the short amount of time that had passed (Figs 1-27a and 1-27b). The blood clot site retained a peripheral erythema and obvious exuberant granulation tissue with only the beginning of an epithelial migration from the periphery. The PRP clot site showed no such ring of erythema and only the remnant of already replaced granulation tissue. The dull sheen of its surface represented a thin layer of epithelium that had already migrated across the entire wound, as documented by the histopathologic sections taken from each site. The normal clot site showed plump young fibroblasts and macrophages with numerous small capillaries typical of an immature wound (Figs 1-28a and 1-28b). The epithelial edge was blunt and showed no obvious migration front. In contrast, the site of the PRP clot showed an obvious front of

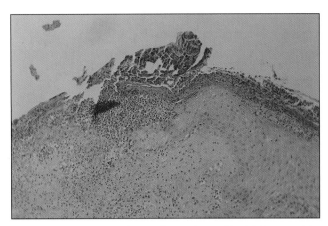

Fig 1-29a Histology from the 6-day split-thickness skin graft donor site enhanced with PRP shows obvious epithelial budding and mature connective tissue development exemplified by spindle-shaped fibroblasts and collagen bundles.

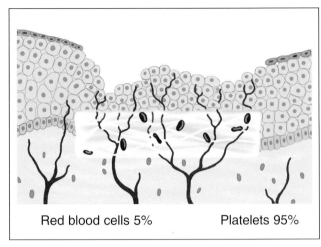

Red blood cells 5%   Platelets 95%

Fig 1-29b Illustration of the histology shown in Fig 1-29a.

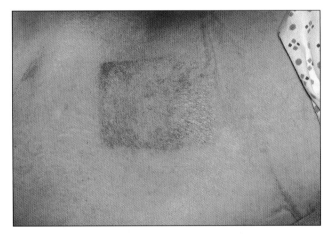

Fig 1-30a At 45 days, a split-thickness skin graft donor site without PRP enhancement features only a thin epithelial layer over a hypervascular connective tissue indicative of immature healing.

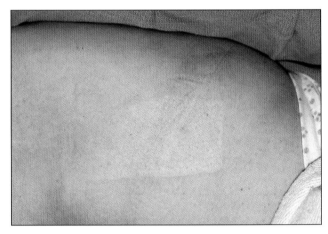

Fig 1-30b At 45 days, a split-thickness skin graft donor site (on the opposite leg of the same individual) enhanced with PRP is more flesh colored, indicating a thicker epithelial covering, and regression of the hypervascular phase, indicating wound maturation.

advancing epithelium over a mature dermis, as evidenced by more spindle-shaped fibroblasts and collagen bundles (Figs 1-29a and 1-29b). The PRP clot site was significantly advanced in its healing rate and maturity as compared to the native blood clot site.

As the skin graft donor site matures, the dermis will develop a reduced vascularity, a reduced fibroblastic cellularity, a normal thickness of epithelium with keratin, and a return of pigment-producing melanocytes. From a clinical perspective, the donor site will progress through a phase of violaceous coloration indicative of a thin epithelial layer over an abundant vascularity. This will fade over 2 to 6 months to become more flesh colored as the epithelium thickens and the hypervascularity of the healing phase regresses to a normal level. In the same study, at

Fig 1-31 The split-thickness skin graft donor sites with and without PRP enhancement shown in Figs 1-27a and 1-27b, now at 6 months. Note the increased scar development and pigment alterations in the site not enhanced with PRP *(left)*.

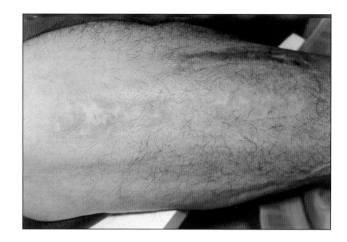

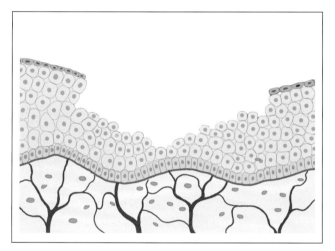

Fig 1-32a Illustration of the split-thickness skin graft donor site without PRP enhancement at 45 days (shown in Fig 1-30a).

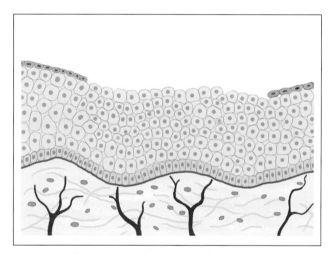

Fig 1-32b Illustration of the split-thickness skin graft donor site with PRP enhancement at 45 days (shown in Fig 1-30b).

45 days the native clot site remained red and numerous small blood vessels could be seen just below the surface (Fig 1-30a). In contrast, at 45 days the PRP clot site was indeed flesh colored and the hypervascularity had obviously regressed, indicative of advanced maturity (Fig 1-30b).

Eventually, all skin graft donor sites heal and develop a certain level of maturity; so what are the advantages of using PRP? They include reduction of pain during the first week and reduction of eventual scarring. Patients reported a 40% reduction in pain at the PRP clot site when comparing separate donor sites on each side of the midline.[12] At 6 months, significant reduction in the scar and wound contraction and improved pigment regeneration were apparent in the PRP-enhanced donor sites when compared to adjacent native blood clot sites (Fig 1-31). The PRP clot site developed less scarring and returned to a more normal skin color by virtue of its earlier epithelial cover of exposed connective tissue and its promotion of melanocyte as well as basal cell regeneration (Figs 1-32a and 1-32b).

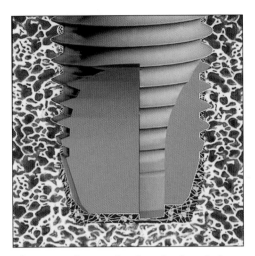

Fig 1-33 When an implant is placed, there is a microgap between the bone and metal surfaces in which a blood clot forms, despite macroscopically implied direct bone-to-metal contact.

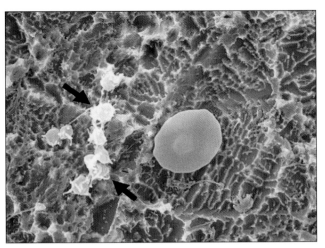

Fig 1-34 Electron micrograph of the microgap around a dental implant showing a red blood cell in the center surrounded by the numerous smaller platelets *(arrows)* with pseudopodial extensions within a fibrin network.

Split-thickness skin grafts were chosen to develop this model of soft tissue healing and its comparison of normal healing to PRP-enhanced healing because they are controlled wounds. However, the mechanism of this healing and how PRP enhances it is applicable to all soft tissue healing. Later chapters will demonstrate PRP enhancement of mucosal flaps, gingival grafts, palatal donor sites, skin graft recipient sites, dermal fat grafts, and facial wounds.

Clinical Effects of PRP on Osseointegration

Osseointegration of dental implants arises from cell migration, differentiation, bone formation, and bone remodeling along the implant surface; each of these processes is platelet- and blood clot–dependent. Therefore, PRP can be be used to enhance osseointegration in patients where osseointegration may be less predictable, such as the elderly and individuals with osteoporosis, diabetes, or other forms of compromised bone regeneration, as well as in the posterior maxilla.

During implant placement, the blood clot, or the PRP that is placed into the drill site, coats the implant surface as well as the microgap (about 25 μm wide) that lies between the actual bone and the metal surface (Fig 1-33). Within this microgap are found the usual components: platelets, red blood cells, white blood cells, and the cell adhesion molecules of fibrin, fibronectin, and vitronectin (Fig 1-34). In this situation the cell adhesion molecules perform the important roles of coating the implant surface and bridging the microgap between the implant surface and the bone (Fig 1-35).

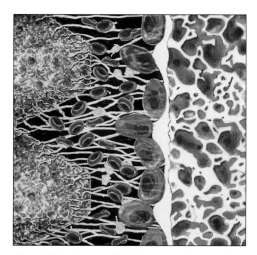

Fig 1-35 The model for osseointegration demonstrates that the implant surface, microgap, and bony wall of the drill site contains fibrin bands connecting the bone to the implant surface, osteoblasts lining the bony walls, and red blood cells and platelets within the microgap.

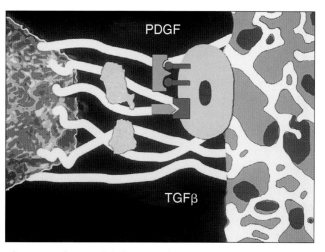

Fig 1-36 The model for osseointegration further demonstrates the degranulation of platelets and their secretion of growth factors that bind to the osteoblast surface membrane to activate a sequence of cell division, migration, osteoid production, bone maturation, and eventual connection of the bony wall to the implant surface.

The model for osseointegration demonstrates that platelets degranulate and secrete their seven growth factors (Fig 1-36). As a result, the osteoblasts and marrow stem cells along the bony walls of the drill site proliferate and migrate along the strands of fibrin and other cell adhesion molecules spanning the microgap (Figs 1-37a to 1-37d). As they migrate along the surface of the fibrin strands, the marrow cells can pull the fibrin strands off the implant surface. (Since fibrin adheres more completely to implants with textured surfaces, they result in more successful osseointegration than the smoother machined-surface implants.) As the marrow cells migrate along the fibrin strands, they undergo differentiation and produce osteoid, a process that has been demonstrated in histologic studies of implant osseointegration (Fig 1-38). This migration, differentiation, and bone-production sequence is often misconceived; the notion that the osteoblast crawls across a rope of fibrin, leaving bone behind it like a snail may leave a slime trail, is inaccurate. In truth, it is more like a chain-link addition type of growth: A migrating stem cell divides and then differentiates into an osteoblast, stops its migration, and secretes osteoid, which then encases the osteoblast, thus turning it into an osteocyte. The daughter cell from the cell division, which was pushed forward toward the implant surface, now itself divides to produce another daughter cell and then undergoes an osteoblastic differentiation and osteoid production to become another osteocyte. This process is repeated until a strut of bone reaches the implant and then begins the same process along the implant surface. The only difference is that it does not occur directly on the metal implant surface but rather on the fibrin that adheres to the metal surface (Figs 1-39a and 1-39b). Once again, understanding this process explains the greater bone-implant contact achieved with textured-surface implants, since fibrin adheres more readily to such surfaces, and underscores the importance of fibrin and other cell adhesion molecules in the process of osseointegration.

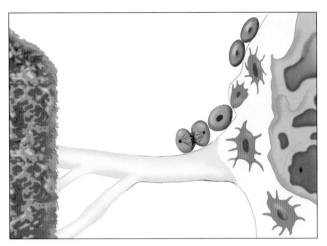

Fig 1-37a Growth factor activation of osteoblasts causes cell divisions along the surface of the fibrin strand.

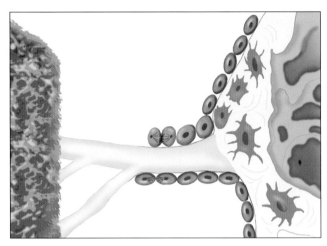

Fig 1-37b As cells divide along the fibrin strand, the lead daughter cell is advanced toward the implant surface and the stationary daughter cell becomes an osteoblast that differentiates further and secretes osteoid.

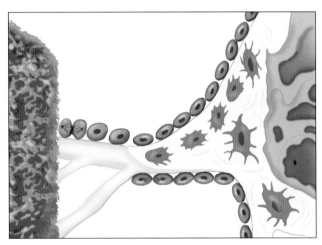

Fig 1-37c As further cell divisions occur, the lead osteoblast daughter cells come into contact with the implant surface, and the trailing daughter cells that secrete osteoid become encased in their mineral matrix to become true osteocytes as a bridge of bone begins to develop toward the implant surface.

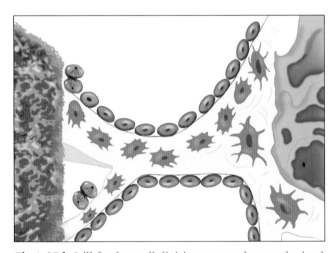

Fig 1-37d Still further cell divisions now advance the lead daughter cell along the implant surface and more trailing osteoblasts mature into osteocytes and form the bridge of osseointegration across the microgap and now along the implant surface itself.

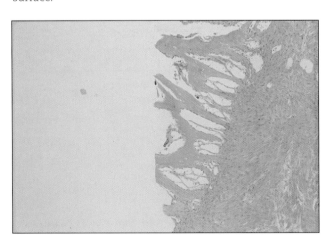

Fig 1-38 Histology of osseointegration confirms the model shown in Figs 1-37a to 1-37d. Note the stem cells to the right forming projections of osteoid toward the now-vacated implant surface on the left. There is osteoblastic rimming on the osteoid projections and encasement of osteoblasts into true osteocytes. Note the remnants of the fibrin bands between the osteoid projections.

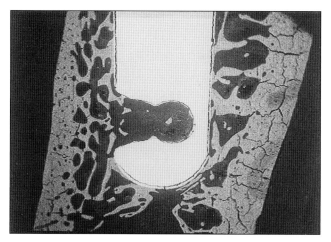

Fig 1-39a Backscatter electron micrograph of an osseo-integrated implant confirms this model of osseointegration and shows bony connections between the endosteal surface of a mandibular cortex to the implant surface and bone formation along the implant surface.

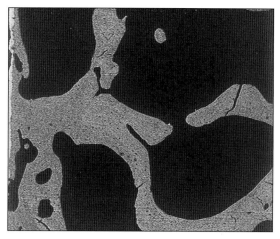

Fig 1-39b High-power view of Fig 1-39a shows the migration of bone along the implant surface and a cement line between the implant surface and the actual bone.

The work by Davies et al has shown that it is not actual bone that comes into direct contact with the metal surface, but rather the natural bone cement commonly seen in the resting or reversal lines of von Ebner.[13] This is similar to the process of new bone remodeling, in which osteoblasts produce a cementing substance against the surface of mature bone to anchor new bone to it and prevent separation (Fig 1-40). Osseointegration relies upon the same cementing substance to anchor new bone to the metal implant surface. While true bone is type I collagen interspersed with calcium hydroxyapatite crystals and trace amounts of growth factors such as BMP and ILG, the cementing substance is sialoprotein and osteopontin with interspersed crystals of calcium hypophosphate (Fig 1-41). This biologic cement flows into the undercuts, grooves, and valleys of the implant surface because it has the consistency of toothpaste and will behave like unset plaster. As the cement sets (ie, crystals of calcium hypophosphate form), the osteoblast embeds collagen fibers into the cement substance as well as its own osteoid; like construction reinforcement rods, these collagen fibers anchor the new bone to the cement (Fig 1-42). Thus, osseointegration is actually a 5-μm-thick cement band adhered to the implant surface into which true bone is anchored. The sequential processes of initial cell proliferation, migration, and differentiation, followed by cement and osteoid secretion, are initiated by and dependent upon the growth factors derived from platelets.

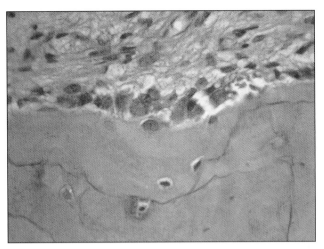

Fig 1-40 The cement line that connects the implant surface to bone is identical to the reversal or resting lines of von Ebner, which are commonly seen in normal bone histology and function physiologically to anchor new bone to old bone and prevent their separation.

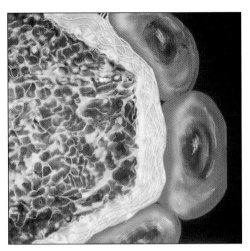

Fig 1-41 The cementing substance that is secreted onto the metal surface is not true bone but the reversal line of von Ebner. This cement is composed of osteopontin and sialoprotein in which crystals of calcium hypophosphate form as the mineral rather than as calcium hydroxyapatite.

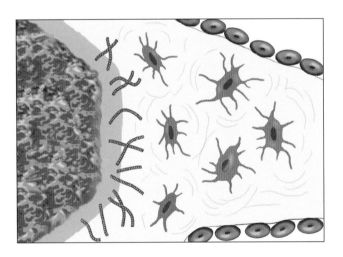

Fig 1-42 Osseointegration is actually bone anchored to the metal surface through the 5-μm-thick cementing substance. True bone is anchored in turn to the cementing substance when the bone embeds collagen fibers into the cementing substance. These collagen fibers perform a function similar to that of reinforced steel rods used in highway construction.

Effects of PRP on Bone Regeneration Using Bone Substitutes

Because the introduction of PRP involved studies documenting the enhancement of autogenous bone and soft tissue regeneration, its benefits were assumed to depend on the presence of autogenous graft cells and therefore to be limited to autogenous grafts. However, recent studies of PRP have shown enhancement of nearly all bone substitute materials as well.[14,15] The reason is that autogenous cells are responsible

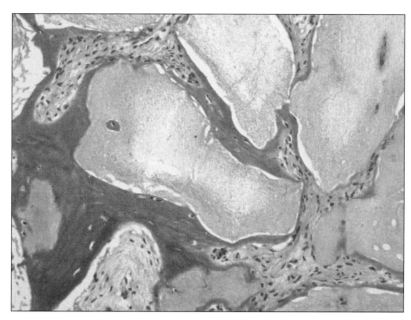

Fig 1-43 Bone regeneration is seen here around the PepGen P-15 (Dentsply Friadent CeraMed) bone substitute particles, and a direct bone-to-particle contact is developed through the secretion of a cementing substance on the bone substitute particle surface so that the bone substitute becomes "osseointegrated." (Courtesy of Dr Paul Petrungaro, Stillwater, Minnesota.)

for new bone formation even when a bone substitute is used. Instead of being transplanted, the autogenous cells migrate into the area of the bone substitute graft to occupy spaces between and around the particles, similar to the mechanism just described for osseointegration. In other words, a bone substitute graft forms new bone via *osteoconduction* from adjacent osteoprogenitor cells, while the autogenous graft forms new bone via *transplantation* of osteoprogenitor cells from a distant site. Certainly an autogenous bone graft places many more osteoprogenitor cells into the graft site and is considered the clinical gold standard. However, reasonable bone regeneration can occur in a bone substitute graft if the material adsorbs fibrin, if its particles are not packed too tightly, and if it supports osteoconduction via either its surface or its porosity (Fig 1-43). Since fewer osteoprogenitor cells are contained in such grafts as compared to autogenous grafts, and since a significant migration is required to fill the graft volume, upregulation of these osteoprogenitor cells and matrix formation for osteoconduction by PRP is even more valuable.

Despite claims to the contrary, no bone substitute or allogeneic bone preparation is truly osteoinductive in humans.[16] Even allogeneic bone, whether mineralized or demineralized, does not contain a sufficient concentration of bioactive BMP to induce new bone in humans. Therefore, all bone substitutes today depend on osteoconduction from host site osteoprogenitor cells to form new bone in the graft. The mechanism by which this occurs can be illustrated in the placement of bone substitutes in the sinus lift graft. In this situation, the particles of a bone substitute material are usually placed within the sinus space below an elevated mem-

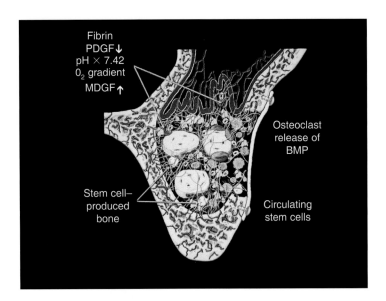

Fig 1-44 A particulate bone substitute graft in the maxillary sinus lift within its biochemical environment of a blood clot, which contains fibrin, fibronectin, vitronectin, red blood cells, and platelets.

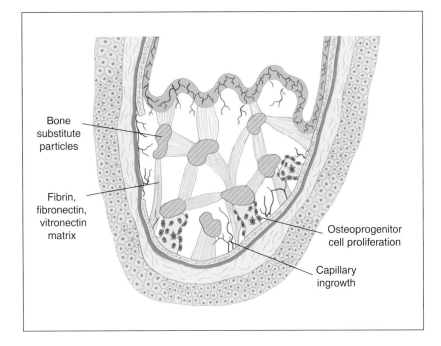

Fig 1-45 Bone regeneration in a bone substitute graft in the maxillary sinus requires capillary ingrowth into the volume space of the graft, osteoprogenitor cell proliferation, and migration from the surrounding bony walls and then actual bone formation around the bone substitute particles.

Fig 1-46 Since a bone substitute graft requires growth factor–related recruitment of osteoprogenitor cells, their migration, eventual bone formation, and then bone maturation, it will require a longer period of time before stable bone with a density capable of implant primary stability develops. Therefore, enhancement with PRP-related growth factors can be of significant value.

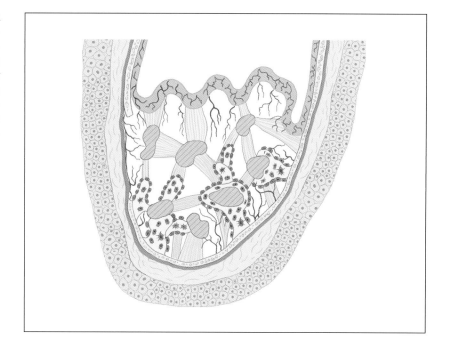

brane. The particles become enmeshed in a blood clot containing fibrin, fibronectin, vitronectin, red blood cells, white blood cells, and the ubiquitous blood platelets (Fig 1-44). If it were a PRP clot, the platelet numbers would be increased four- to sevenfold. Within 10 minutes of clotting, the platelets degranulate and secrete their seven growth factors. Some of these growth factors act on the severed blood vessels of the bony walls and undersurface of the sinus membrane to induce a capillary ingrowth into the graft volume, while others act on the medial and lateral bony walls as well as the sinus floor to initiate the migration, differentiation, and bone production sequence already elucidated in osseointegration (Fig 1-45). As demonstrated in the model for osseointegration, these osteoprogenitor cells migrate along the fibrin network that bridges the gaps between bone and bone substitute particles and between one bone substitute particle and another (see Fig 1-43). Fibrin adheres to the bone substitute particles; osteoprogenitor cells then migrate along the fibrin surface to form a cementing substance and produce bone. Thus, like the hydroxyapatite coating on some dental implants, the bone substitute particles actually become osseointegrated. The network of bone forms around these particles and interconnects to at least one native bony wall to form a stable graft (Fig 1-46). Since the steps leading to bone formation include growth factor recruitment and stimulation of cells, their migration, and differentiation before bone is actually formed (as compared to an autogenous graft, where many already differentiated cells are present in large numbers), bone formation in bone substitute grafts takes longer and forms less total bone. PRP has the ability to stimulate more bone formation in a shorter time when used in conjunction with a bone substitute graft.

References

1. Knighton DR, Silver IA, Hunt TK. Regulation of wound-healing angiogenesis: Effect of oxygen gradients and inspired oxygen concentration. Surgery 1981;90:262–270.

2. Knighton DR, Hunt TK, Scheuenstuhl H, Halliday BJ, Werb Z, Banda MJ. Oxygen tension regulates the expression of angiogenesis factor by macrophages. Science 1983;221: 1283–1285.

3. Hunt TK. The physiology of wound healing. Ann Emerg Med 1988;17:1265–1273

4. Marx RE, Johnson RP. Studies in the radiobiology of osteoradionecrosis and their clinical significance. Oral Surg Oral Med Oral Pathol 1982;64:379–390.

5. Marx RE, Ehler WJ, Tayapongsak PT, Pierce LW. Relationship of oxygen dose to angiogenesis induction in irradiated tissue. Am J Surg 1990;160:519–524.

6. Cordeiro PG, Disa JJ, Hidalgo DA, Hu QY. Reconstruction of the mandible with osseous free flaps: A 10-year experience with 150 consecutive patients. Plast Reconstr Surg 1999;104: 1314–1320.

7. Marx RE, Smith BR. An improved technique for development of the pectoralis major myocutaneous flap. J Oral Maxillofac Surg 1990;48:1168–1180.

8. Davis JC, Hunt TK (eds). Problem Wounds—The Role of Oxygen. New York: Elsevier, 1988.

9. Knighton DR, Hunt TK, Thakeral KK, Goodsen WH III. Role of platelets and fibrin in the healing sequence: An in vivo study of angiogenesis and collagen synthesis. Ann Surg 1982; 196:379–388.

10. Caplan AI. Mesenchymal stem cells and gene therapy. Clin Orthop 2000;379(suppl): S67–S70.

11. Marx RE, Carlson ER, Eichstaedt RM, Schimmele SR, Strauss JE, Georgeff KR. Platelet rich plasma: Growth factor enhancement for bone grafts. Oral Surg Oral Med Oral Pathol Oral Radiol Endod 1998;85:638–646.

12. Marx RE. Platelet-rich plasma: Evidence to support its use. J Oral Maxillofac Surg 2004;62: 489–496.

13. Davies JE, Lowenberg B, Shiga A. The bone-titanium interface in vitro. J Biomed Mater Res 1990;24:1289–1306.

14. Kassolis JD, Rosen PS, Reynolds MA. Alveolar ridge and sinus augmentation utilizing platelet-rich plasma in combination with freeze-dried bone allograft: Case series. J Periodontol 2000;71:1654–1661.

15. Camargo PM, Lekovic V, Weinlaender M, Vasilic N, Madzarevic M, Kenney EB. Platelet-rich plasma and bovine porous bone mineral combined with guided tissue regeneration in the treatment of intrabony defects in humans. J Periodontal Res 2002;37:300–306.

16. Garg AK. Grafting materials in repair and restoration. In: Lynch SE, Genco RJ, Marx RE (eds). Tissue Engineering: Applications in Maxillofacial Surgery and Periodontics. Chicago: Quintessence, 1999:83–101.

Development of Platelet-Rich Plasma and Its Clinical Importance

Not all platelet-rich plasma (PRP) is the same. The preceding chapter should have given the reader a sufficient understanding of the biology of platelets to appreciate that effective PRP should concentrate viable bioactive platelets and that their secretion of growth factors is dependent on the clotting process. This chapter focuses on how PRP is developed clinically so that the reader can use it effectively and choose the best PRP processing device for his or her practice or particular type of surgery.

The Early Days of PRP

PRP has been available for less than a decade. In the early 1990s, PRP could only be developed by means of a cell separator or plasmapheresis machine (Fig 2-1). These devices were as large as a kitchen stove, expensive ($40,000 in 1996), and costly to operate (about $300 for a disposable canister and a dedicated operator or perfusionist). They were, however, effective in separating autologous blood into its three basic components: red blood cells, the combined white blood cell and platelet layer (known as the *buffy coat*), and plasma (Fig 2-2). At that time, nearly a full unit of blood (450 mL) was needed and was usually obtained through a central venous line. Therefore, the early use of PRP was confined to the operating room, primarily for large-scale surgeries.

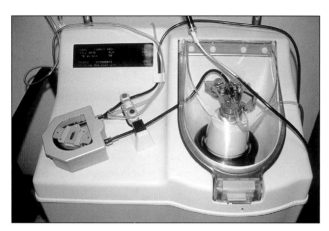

Fig 2-1 Plasmapheresis/cell separator receiving autologous blood from a central venous access with pump advancing 450 mL of blood into centrifugation bowl.

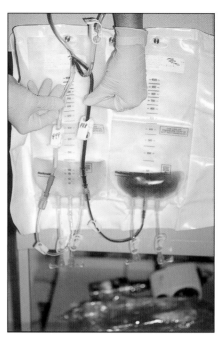

Fig 2-2 Attendant (doctor, nurse, or perfusionist) directing separation of PRP component and platelet-poor plasma (PPP) component. Note the red blood cells remained in the centrifugation bowl and could be reinfused.

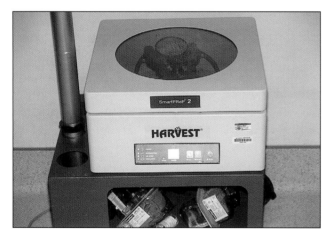

Fig 2-3 This fully automated office device, which also can be used as an in-patient hospital device, has been cleared by the US Food and Drug Administration (FDA). It uses 120, 60, or as little as 20 mL of autologous blood (Harvest Technologies).

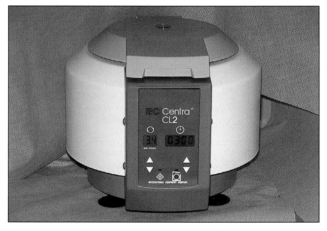

Fig 2-4 FDA-cleared semi-automated office and in-patient hospital device uses 60 mL of autologous blood (Implant Innovations Inc).

A growing demand for PRP, first by dental specialists[1–3] and, more recently, by facial cosmetic surgeons[4,5] and wound care centers[6] led to the development of smaller, more compact office-based devices that required smaller quantities of the patient's blood. These devices have gained wide acceptance in outpatient surgeries and have even replaced many of the cell separators in the operating room (Figs 2-3 and 2-4).

Fig 2-5 At its base, the cephalic vein *(arrow)* is one of the larger diameter and most stable veins in the hand-wrist region for phlebotomy.

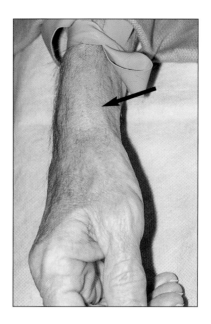

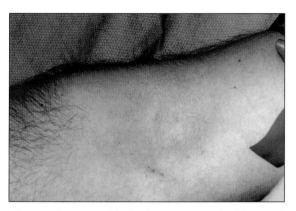

Fig 2-6 The antecubital veins represent the ideal and most commonly used phlebotomy site due to their stability and large diameter.

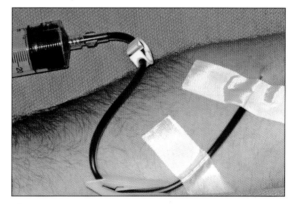

Fig 2-7 As the blood is drawn, the anticoagulant ACD-A already in the syringe immediately binds blood calcium to inhibit clotting.

Principles of Platelet Separation and Concentration

Platelet separation and concentration starts with an aseptic and minimally traumatic phlebotomy technique for the withdrawal of a small volume of blood appropriate for the particular device to be used, usually 20 to 60 mL. A 19-gauge needle or larger should be used to avoid platelet disruption or activation in the lumen of a narrow needle. A large vein such as the wrist vein over the radius (ie, the beginning of the cephalic vein) (Fig 2-5) or an antecubital vein (Fig 2-6) should be chosen. So that the blood is immediately coagulated, the syringe should contain anticoagulant citrate dextrose A (ACD-A) (Fig 2-7). Ethylenediaminetetraacetic acid (EDTA), which is used in diagnostic blood laboratories, is not recommended

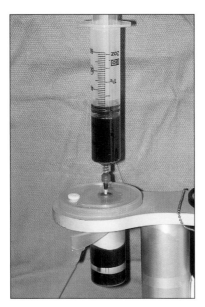

Fig 2-8 The anticoagulated blood is placed into the receiving chamber marked by the red top prior to placing it into the centrifugation device.

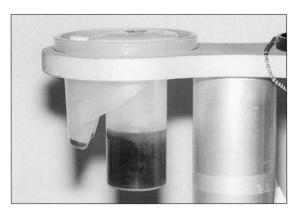

Fig 2-9 After PRP separation, the residual red blood cells are seen here in the chamber to the right, while the chamber to the left shows a red blood cell "button" at the bottom, a thin buffy coat layer just above, and the clear yellow platelet-poor plasma. The concentrated platelets are located in the red blood cell button, the buffy coat, and the bottommost few milliliters of the plasma fraction.

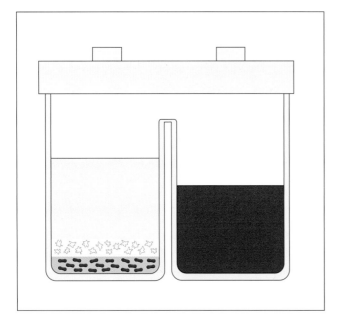

Fig 2-10 The separation spin already separated the red blood cells from the plasma, platelets, and white blood cells. Here the concentration spin has consolidated the platelet–white blood cell concentrate at the bottom of the second chamber; it is seen layered above a small amount of residual red blood cells and overlayed by PPP.

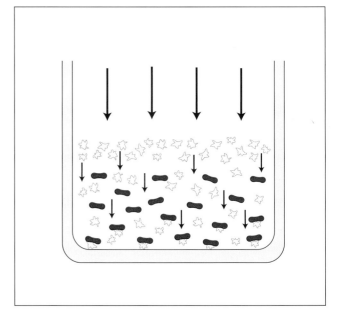

Fig 2-11 The concave-convex shape of red blood cells can entrap platelets during centrifugation. This is one reason why single-spin devices and poorly designed PRP machines often produce poor platelet yields and subtherapeutic levels of growth factors.

for this purpose because it is damaging to platelet membranes. Citrate phosphate dextrose (CPD), which is used to store red blood cells, also is not recommended for this purpose because it does not support platelet metabolism as well as ACD-A. Today, blood banks use only ACD-A as a platelet-preserving solution for platelet transfusion.

When 20 mL of autologous blood is used, 2 mL of ACD-A should be placed in the syringe prior to blood withdrawal. When 60 mL of autologous blood is drawn, 7 mL of ACD-A should be used. Using the SmartPReP device by Harvest Technologies, the anticoagulated autologous blood is placed into the red-topped canister, which is then placed into the device (Fig 2-8). Although all PRP processing devices operate by centrifugation, only a few produce consistently high concentrations of viable bioactive platelets. Effective platelet separation and concentration are a product of gravitational forces (g forces) over time, usually measured in minutes (g minutes). To separate and concentrate platelets, the device must use two separate centrifugations, called *spins*. The first spin, known as the *separation spin*, separates the red blood cells from the rest of the whole blood (white blood cells, platelets, and plasma). This is followed by a *concentration spin*, which separates and compacts the platelets, white blood cells, and a small number of residual red blood cells from the plasma after 95% or more of the red blood cells have been separated and sequestered into another compartment of the canister (Figs 2-9 and 2-10).

Single-spin machines are incapable of separating and concentrating platelets to a therapeutic level. Because of the convex-concave shape of the red blood cell and the relatively smaller size of the platelets, the smaller platelets get trapped in the concavity of the larger red blood cells and become compacted with them rather than being concentrated separately (Fig 2-11).

The most effective PRP development occurs when a separation spin of about 1,000 g for 4 minutes (4,000 g minutes) is followed by a concentration spin of about 800 g for 8 to 9 minutes (6,400 to 7,200 g minutes) for a total of about 11,000 g minutes. This force application is about one third the value known to disrupt platelet cell membranes (30,000 g minutes).

Some authors and manufacturers tout the revolutions per minute (RPMs) of a particular device; however, RPMs have no direct relationship to PRP development. Their role, along with the shape of the container, is to control the g forces on the platelets. Each of the two spins must be timed precisely to gain consistent platelet separation and concentration. This is best accomplished by a fully automated device that avoids manual manipulations that can disrupt the platelet separation. In addition, the effectiveness of the device should be wholly independent of the patient's hematocrit. In fully automated systems, this is usually accomplished by a density-dependent floating shelf; in systems that are less automated, this is accomplished by the more work intensive but equally effective manual separation of the red blood cell fraction after the separation spin.

After the completion of the concentration spin, a few residual red blood cells, along with nearly all of the white blood cells and platelets, will be compacted at the bottom of the PRP compartment and overlaid by a volume of plasma (see Fig 2-9). Together, these will appear as a small layer of red blood cells surrounded by a thin white line (the so-called buffy coat) over a larger volume of straw-

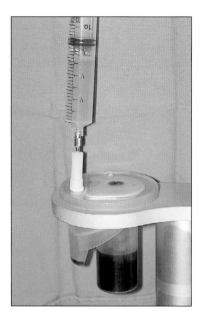

Fig 2-12 A fixed amount of PPP is aspirated, leaving a residual 7- or 10-mL volume of plasma and the platelet concentrate.

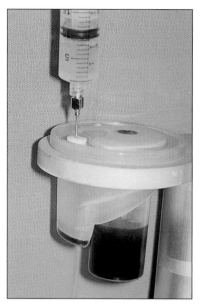

Fig 2-13a The residual volume of plasma is aspirated and will then be squirted back along the side walls and bottom of the canister to suspend the platelet concentrate. This maneuver is performed three times. The subsequent suspension is true PRP.

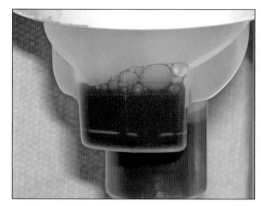

Fig 2-13b Resuspension of the concentrated platelets into PRP is accomplished by ejecting the residual PPP down the walls of the canister three times.

colored but mostly clear liquid, which is the plasma. Commonly described as a *red blood cell button*, this appearance of the PRP as it emerges from the machine is a sign of quality for the clinician. The younger platelets, which contain more growth factors, are larger and therefore centrifuge out in the upper layer of the red blood cell fraction. The red blood cell button indicates the presence of these younger and more complete platelets.

After the platelets are separated and concentrated in the canister, and the canister is removed from the machine, the PRP is not yet fully developed. A specific amount of the plasma layer is aspirated away; this is the PPP (Fig 2-12). For the SmartPReP device, the remaining small volume of plasma is then used to resuspend the concentrated platelets. This is accomplished by drawing up the remaining plasma volume into the syringe without the stopper ring and then ejecting it down the walls and onto the bottom of the canister three times (Figs 2-13a and 2-13b). Following this maneuver, the suspension of concentrated platelets, which now contains a small number of red blood cells and white blood cells in plasma and usually appears as a light red suspension, is the developed PRP (Fig 2-14).

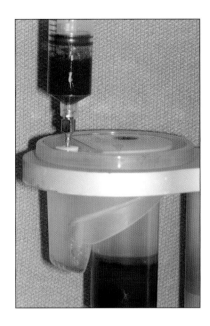

Fig 2-14 The aspirate suspension of PRP is ready for activation and will remain sterile with viable and active platelets for up to 8 hours.

Unnecessary terminology confusion

PRP has been described in the literature under several different names and abbreviations: autologous platelet concentrate (APC or APC+), platelet concentrate (PC),[7] platelet gel (PG),[5] plasma-rich growth factors (PRGF)[8] (this one is not only backwards but absurdly incorrect), and derivations of the latter—plasma very rich in growth factors (PVRGF) and plasma very, very rich in growth factors (PVVRGF)[8]—which are simply ludicrous.

As the preceding discussion should have made clear, platelets are first separated and then concentrated, and therefore it might seem reasonable to use the term *autologous platelet concentrate* or simply *platelet concentrate*. However, the usable biologic product is derived only when this platelet concentrate is resuspended in a small volume of plasma. Therefore, *platelet-rich plasma* (PRP) is the most accurate term to describe what is used on an actual patient. PRP is not a gel; a gel is a colloid formed by chemically treating or heat-treating proteins, whereas PRP is a clot. Of course, *plasma-rich growth factors* is overtly wrong because it is not the plasma that is concentrated into the platelets, but the platelets that are concentrated into a small volume of plasma, which then release their growth factors. Derivations of this as *plasma very rich in growth factors and plasma very, very rich in growth factors* are equally wrong and merely betray the self-serving motives of the authors who coined them.[8]

Such terms are sometimes used interchangeably in presentations and literature and serve only to confuse the audience. In addition, their purpose may be to disguise a platelet preparation that is not the biologic or clinical equivalent of the PRP that has a proven clinical outcome.

Storage and Activation of PRP

Developed PRP is anticoagulated and will remain in that state until a clotting process is initiated. PRP has been found to remain sterile and its platelets to remain viable and bioactive for up to 8 hours when stored at room temperature.[9] Therefore, it is recommended that the PRP remain anticoagulated until it is needed at the tissue site. Because it can be stored for up to 8 hours, the PRP will be effective even when used during a long procedure or when the procedure is delayed. However, storing PRP for more than 8 hours is not recommended since its viability has not been tested beyond that time frame, and refrigeration and/or freezing without cryopreservatives disrupts platelet membranes. Since the development of PRP requires only a small amount of blood, and the entire process can be completed in just 15 minutes or less, it is best to discard any unused PRP after 8 hours and develop a second batch of PRP.

The ACD-A that is used as an anticoagulant in developing PRP inhibits clotting by binding calcium. Therefore, activation of the PRP requires replacement of calcium and initiation of the cascade of blood coagulation. This can be accomplished by adding 5 mL of a 10% calcium chloride ($CaCl_2$) solution to 5,000 units of topical bovine thrombin (Fig 2-15). When used in very small volumes, this solution will clot the PRP into what is often termed a *smart clot*. To clinically apply PRP, the anticoagulated PRP solution is placed into a 10-mL syringe and the $CaCl_2$-thrombin solution is placed into a l-mL syringe (ie, a tuberculin syringe). The two syringes are then placed into an ejection assembly that has a nozzle to combine the two solutions into what looks like a squirt gun (Fig 2-16). Upon pushing the lever of the injection assembly, each solution is expressed in a proportion of 10:1 through the nozzle tip, which delivers the PRP to a precise location, and clotting occurs within 6 to 10 seconds. Alternatively, the PRP can be activated in its cup receptacle by adding just two drops of the $CaCl_2$-thrombin solution to it and then carrying the activated PRP clot to the tissue site (Figs 2-17a and 2-17b). Another option is to aspirate the anticoagulated PRP into a syringe and then to aspirate the equivalent of two drops of the $CaCl_2$-thrombin solution into the syringe, along with a small amount of air to be used as a mixing bubble. In 6 to 10 seconds, the clotted (activated) PRP can be expressed onto the tissue site (Fig 2-18). It is important to note that using more than 2 drops of the $CaCl_2$-thrombin solution is counterproductive. A larger volume of this solution will not speed the clotting process but will actually slow it down or inhibit clotting altogether by diluting the fibrinogen concentration, which is the rate-limiting factor in clot formation.

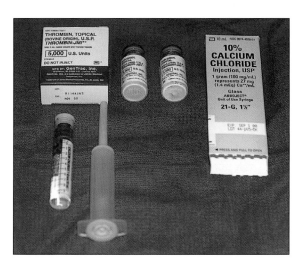

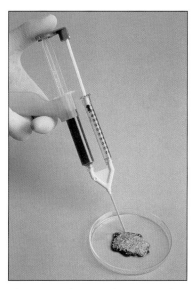

Fig 2-15 PRP must be activated by the clotting process. Therefore, 5 mL of a 10% calcium chloride solution is added to 5,000 units of lyophilized bovine thrombin as the ideal clot initiator.

Fig 2-16 The ejection assembly mixes the PRP with the CaCl$_2$-thrombin solution at a 10:1 ratio so that clotting takes place in 6 seconds or less.

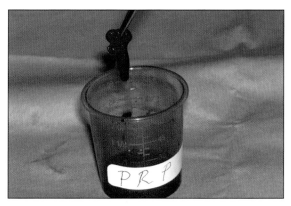

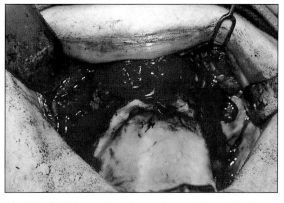

Fig 2-17a An activated PRP clot has sufficient texture to be picked up with a forceps and transferred to the recipient site.

Fig 2-17b When placed on the surface of a bone graft, activated PRP will seep its growth factors down into the graft and also into the covering periosteum or mucosa.

Fig 2-18 PRP can also be activated in a syringe and ejected directly onto the recipient site.

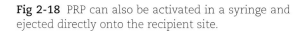

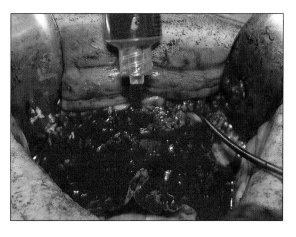

PRP constructs

Several PRP constructs can be used by the clinical surgeon. One of the most common constructs is formed by applying the PRP clot to the graft, which will consolidate bone substitute particles, particulate allogeneic bone, and/or autogenous cancellous bone marrow particles together into a workable complex with improved handling properties (Figs 2-19 to 2-21). Another recommended use is to place one or several layers of clotted PRP over a bone graft (see Fig 2-17b), an access window of a sinus lift surgery (Fig 2-22), or a membrane. This allows the growth factors to seep out of the clot and soak into both the graft and the overlying soft tissue, thereby enhancing the healing of both. Another construct of PRP is a PRP membrane, which can be formed by expressing a 1- to 3-mL pool of PRP onto a smooth surface (Fig 2-23). Once the PRP clots (6 to 10 seconds) and matures (1 minute), it can be picked up with a spatula-like instrument and applied in the same manner as any other short-term membrane (eg, a collagen membrane, which lasts for about 5 to 7 days) (Figs 2-24 and 2-25). Other applications include the incubation of bone[10] and soft tissue grafts in anticoagulated PRP for several minutes and the rehydration of freeze-dried allogeneic bone[6] or dermis (AlloDerm [LifeCell]). These grafts and tissues are then coated with the $CaCl_2$-thrombin solution immediately before placement to activate the PRP. Applications of PRP are limited only by the understanding and inventiveness of the surgeon.

Unnecessary concerns about bovine thrombin

Because it is an autogenous preparation, PRP is completely free of any transmissible human diseases such as HIV, hepatitis, West Nile fever, and Creutzfeldt-Jakob disease (CJD; also commonly referred to as *mad cow disease*).[11] It is therefore also accepted well by patients. Specifically related to CJD, concerns have been advanced about the use of bovine thrombin as the clot initiator. The transmission vector of CJD is a prion (ie, a small self-replicating protein) that to date has been found only in neural tissues of the central nervous system in cattle, sheep, cats, humans, etc, whereas bovine thrombin is derived exclusively from blood and is then heat processed for purification. Moreover, bovine thrombin has a completely negative history of CJD in more than 10 million uses in diverse surgeries worldwide. It remains in standard use today in many surgeries and is the safe initiator of clotting for the development of PRP.

A more rational clinical concern relates to the rare cases in which bovine thrombin was used as a hemostatic agent in open orthopedic, neurosurgical, and cardiovascular surgeries that later developed bleeding episodes.[12,13] Fewer than 20 such cases have been reported, and each of these adverse events has been thoroughly investigated. The second-set bleeding episodes in these patients was due to antibodies not against bovine or human thrombin but against bovine factor Va, which was a contaminant in certain commercial preparations of bovine thrombin.[14,15] These antibodies cross-reacted with human factor Va and produced coagulopathies as well as the rare bleeding episodes. Since 1997, the processing of bovine thrombin by GenTrac (Jones Medical Industries) has virtually eliminated contamination of bovine thrombin with bovine factor Va. Prior to 1997, levels of

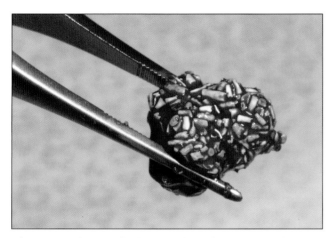

Fig 2-19a A bone substitute–activated PRP composite contains growth factors and the fibrin-fibronectin-vitronectin matrix between them.

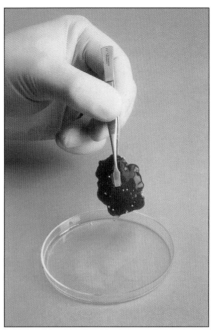

Fig 2-19b Activated PRP congeals bone substitute particles as well as autogenous and allogeneic bone particles for an easy-to-place composite.

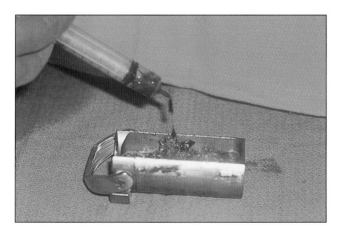

Fig 2-20 PRP may also be activated without using the ejection assembly. Here the PRP was aspirated into a 5-mL syringe, after which less than 0.25 mL of the $CaCl_2$-thrombin solution was aspirated and mixed by turning the syringe.

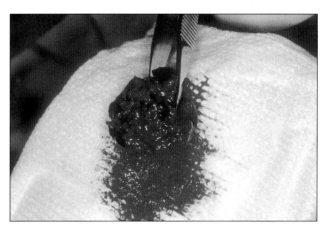

Fig 2-21 PRP added to autogenous bone creates improved handling properties of the graft material.

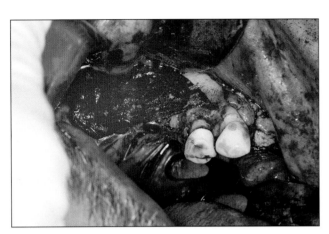

Fig 2-22 Activated PRP placed over a sinus lift window.

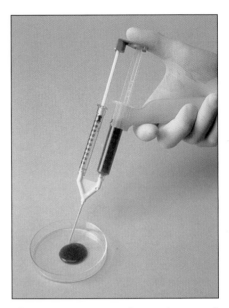

Fig 2-23 A PRP membrane is started by activating a 3-cm-diameter pool of PRP on a smooth sterile surface.

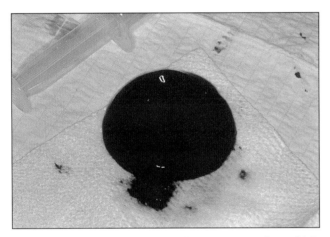

Fig 2-24 A PRP membrane requires a mature clot, which takes about 60 seconds to develop.

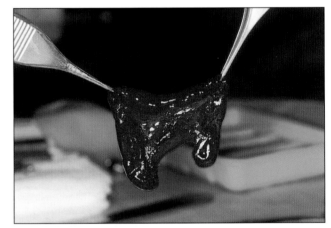

Fig 2-25 A mature PRP membrane can be used in the same manner as any fast-resorbing collagen membrane. However, it is essentially an autologous fibrin membrane that also contains the seven growth factors from the platelets plus the cell adhesion molecules vitronectin and fibronectin.

bovine factor Va in bovine thrombin reached 50 mg/mL; today they are less than 0.2 mg/mL, and no further cases related to this specific preparation have been reported.[11,12] In addition, the bovine thrombin preparations used in the cases reported were high in dosage (more than 10,000 units) and were applied directly to open wounds, where absorption into the systemic circulation is certain. The use of bovine thrombin in PRP is low in dosage (less than 200 units), is topical (does not enter the systemic circulation), and is already clotted when it comes into contact with human tissues. It is therefore not absorbed systemically but instead is subsequently engulfed and digested by the macrophages that also digest the clot itself.

Today, bovine thrombin prepared by adding 5 mL of a 10% $CaCl_2$ solution to the lyophilized bovine thrombin preparation is the standard for initiating clotting of PRP and activating the platelets. It will lead to rapid clotting (within 6 to 10 seconds) and form a cross-linked clot that will allow for convenient handling and the binding of particulate grafts.

Does PRP promote infections?

The empirical belief that PRP can promote infections is based on the flawed logic that PRP is a blood clot, and blood agar is used in microbiology labs to culture bacteria. PRP is identical in substrate to the blood clot that forms in every wound, and therefore it cannot support bacterial growth any more than any other blood clot. In fact, PRP has a pH of 6.5 to 6.7, whereas a mature blood clot has a pH of 7.0 to 7.2 and therefore may even inhibit bacterial growth, as do other acidic solutions. Therefore, there is the counterbelief that PRP actually inhibits bacterial growth due to its lower pH. On this question, no clear studies or data are available. Based on our experience in comparing similar types of bone grafts and skin wounds with and without PRP, no differences in the promotion or inhibition of infection complications have been found; each has an incidence of 2.0% to 3.5%. However, the clinician should take heed that preparation of PRP requires the use of an aseptic technique. Several of the PRP development devices that have not been cleared by the FDA do not employ complete sterile or pyrogen-free disposable materials and often use standard laboratory centrifuges, which require numerous sterile barrier punctures that may increase the risk of contamination by the operator.

Which Office PRP Device Is Best?

This chapter has so far established the principles and techniques to develop consistently high platelet yields by centrifugation. However, in selecting a PRP machine, the individual surgeon is not likely to know its g-minute parameters, the outcome of any platelet viability testing, and whether it is a single- or double-spin device. Following are the key features that characterize effective PRP machines:

Table 2-1	Processing Details of Systems Evaluated					
System	Amount of anticoagulated blood (mL)	Sterile barrier entries	No. of processing steps	Operator time (min)	Processing time (min)	Total time (min)
SmartPReP (n = 25)	60	5	4	2	13	15
PCCS (n = 25)	60	5	24	15	17	32
Secquire (n = 5)	50	6	12	10	12	22
CATS (n = 5)	450	4	16	10	10	20
Access (n = 5)	60	3	15	10	15	25
GPS (n = 6)	60	7	23	15	12	27
Magellan (n = 11)	60	2	23	7	16	23

1. **FDA clearance.** The FDA is responsible for reviewing the safety and efficacy of all biologics and devices designed for medical use. For the surgeon's own assurance and medicolegal protection, the use of an FDA-cleared device is strongly recommended. As of this writing, the following PRP devices have been cleared by the FDA:
   - GPS Platelet Separation Kit; Biomet
   - PCCS Graft Delivery System; Implant Innovations Incorporated (3i)
   - Secquire Cell Separator; Perfusion Partners
   - AutoloGel Process Centrifuge; Cytomedix
   - CATS Continuous Autotransfusion System; Fresenius HemoCare
   - Access Sequestration System; Interpore Cross
   - Magellan Autologous Platelet Separator; Medtronic
   - SmartPReP Platelet Concentrate System; Harvest Technologies
2. **Complete or nearly complete automation** (Table 2-1).
3. **Consistent platelet concentration yield of 4 to 6 times baseline per 6-mL volume (approximately 1 million platelets/mL).** This remains the key feature for the clinician to look for in a device, since the more platelets recovered by the PRP device, the more growth factors there will be to enhance healing. A graph of assayed growth factor PDGFab versus the number of platelets (Fig 2-26) clearly shows a linear correlation between growth factor release and the number of platelets. This was also documented in the seminal work by Haynesworth et al,[16] which tested the population growth of mesenchymal stem cells with different concentrations of platelets; several non–platelet-containing solutions served as controls. As shown in Fig 2-27, the controls failed to produce a population growth of the mesenchymal stem cells. However, the response to increasing concentrations of platelets showed an exponential pop-

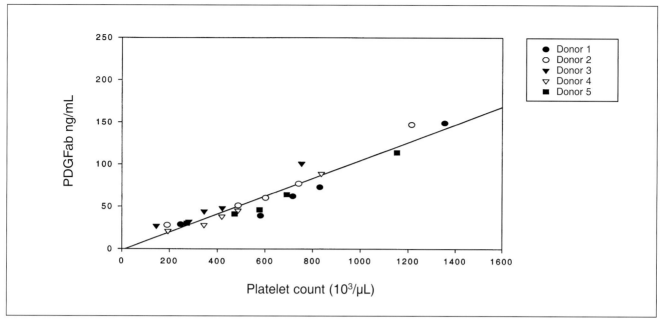

Fig 2-26 PDGFab release with thrombin.

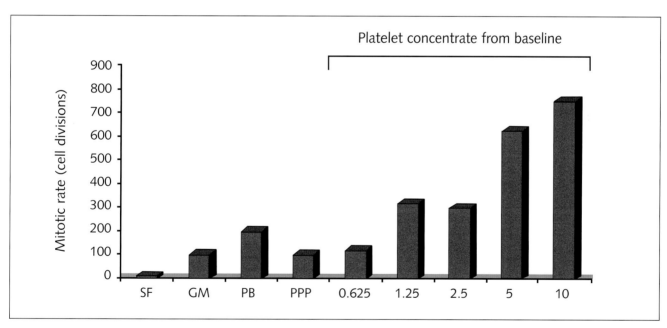

Fig 2-27 Dose-dependent mitogenic effects of platelet-rich releasate on human mesenchymal stem cells. Statistical differences (two-tailed paired t-tests) are shown relative to human mesenchymal stem cell growth medium (GM control) ($P > .005$). (SF, serum-free; GM, growth medium; PB, phosphate buffer.) (Reprinted with permission from Haynesworth et al.[16])

Table 2-2	In Vitro Indicators of Platelet Viability		
	P-selectin (%) (normal 10–20)		Aggregation (%) (normal 81 ± 12)
System	Without ADP	With ADP	With collagen
SmartPReP	13 ± 8	36 ± 12	80 ± 9
PCCS	16 ± 10	37 ± 9	78 ± 7
CATS	9 ± 3	31 ± 2	82 ± 9
Access	43 ± 27	42 ± 14	17 ± 21

ADP = adenosine diphosphate

ulation growth that begins at about 3 times the baseline platelet level and becomes significant at 4 to 5 times baseline. The value at 10 times baseline, which is beyond the capacity of any currently available device, showed an even greater mesenchymal stem cell population growth, indicating that current devices need to be capable of maximum platelet concentration and implying that even further healing enhancement may be possible in the future.

4. **Maintenance of platelet viability and activity after processing.** Platelet viability is measured by the P-selectin test. P-selectin is a protein found in the membrane of the platelet alpha granules. The test measures the P-selectin both prior to and following activation with adenosine diphosphate (ADP). Following platelet activation and fusion of the alpha granule membrane to the platelet cell membrane, detection of the P-selectin on the platelet surface indicates a viable platelet that is capable of degranulation. The P-selectin values of freshly prepared PRP are about 10% to 20% and increase to 40% to 60% following ADP activation. P-selectin values that do not increase with the addition of ADP indicate damaged platelets (Table 2-2).

An alternative measure of platelet viability and activity can be carried out using 200 mg/mL collagen solution to stimulate platelet aggregation. An optical aggregometer can then quantitate the percentage of platelets that aggregate, which is an indicator of both platelet viability and activity. Normal platelet viability and activity values as determined by this method are 81% ± 12%. Values lower than 60% indicate inactive nonsecretory platelets (see Table 2-2).

5. **Amount of autologous blood required (120 mL or less).** Data developed by Sherwin V. Kevy, MD, and May S. Jacobson of the Children's Hospital, Center for Blood Research Laboratories (Harvard Medical School, Boston, MA) using volunteer blood for PRP development in the most commonly used devices provide useful comparisons related to the time required to develop the PRP,

Table 2-3	Comparison of the Platelet Products				
System	Baseline platelet count $\times 10^3/\mu L$	Platelet concentrate volume (mL)	Platelet concentrate count $\times 10^3/\mu L$	Platelet yield (%)	Coefficient of variance (%)
SmartPReP	251 ± 55	9.3 ± 1.8	1016 ± 389	72 ± 10	13
PCCS	268 ± 59	8.2 ± 1.2	1036 ± 446	58 ± 22	38
Secquire	220 ± 13	9.0 ± 0.5	348 ± 194	31 ± 15	48
CATS	239 ± 46	29.0 ± 0.6	992 ± 162	31 ± 5	16
Access	582 ± 128	23.0 ± 0.6	356 ± 233	27 ± 22	81

the blood volume required, the platelet yield, and the platelet viability. These data are presented in Tables 2-1, 2-2, and 2-3.

Table 2-1 lists two devices that require a 450-mL blood draw, making them impractical for office or outpatient surgical use. It also reveals that all but two devices require more than 15 steps for processing, each step inviting the possibility of human error or contamination. Obviously, devices requiring the fewest steps and/or maneuvers to develop the PRP are preferred. Table 2-1 also shows that only two devices require less than 10 minutes of operator time; this is time when the nurse or ancillary personnel is not directly assisting the surgeon or otherwise preparing for the case. Devices that require minimal operator time allow the surgical staff to focus on the surgery itself, and they do not delay a procedure. The time investment can also be compounded by a lengthy processing cycle; this is time when the blood is in the device and the surgeon, nurse, or ancillary personnel can be directly attending to the patient, and therefore it is of less concern. Table 2-1 lists one device with an excessively prolonged operating time. The SmartPReP and the Magellan list the best overall processing characteristics.

Table 2-2 relates comparison data of platelet viability and activity once developed into PRP. These values are important because the platelets are of no biologic or clinical value if they are not viable and capable of secreting their growth factors. This table indicates that all devices except the Access device maintain good platelet viability and activity. Platelets are reasonably hardy to centrifugal forces. If a device produces a high platelet yield and concentration, it can be expected to provide the bioactive growth factors that can enhance wound healing. The low viability and activity of platelets by the Access device may be attributed to mechanical disruption or heat exposure during the processing.

Table 2-3 lists the important features of platelet concentration, platelet yield (the percentage of total available platelets recovered), and the reproducibility and uniformity of the platelet yield (coefficient of variance). This table shows that the SmartPReP and the PCCS were significantly superior in platelet concentration and platelet yield. Both devices yielded over 1 million platelets/µL in a standard volume of 60 mL, which is the clinical benchmark for wound healing enhancement, and both demonstrated a platelet recovery of more than 55%. The CATS device produced a reasonable platelet concentration just below 1 million platelets/µL. The SmartPReP and the CATS devices produced a consistent and uniform product, as demonstrated by their coefficients of variance, which were a low 13% and 16%, respectively. However, the CATS device was inefficient in recovering a high percentage of platelets (only 31%) and its platelet concentrations were obtained only by virtue of the large volume of blood required by this device (450 mL). Therefore, the SmartPReP and PCCS devices seem best suited for office use and/or outpatient surgical practices.

From the composite data presented in the three accompanying tables, the SmartPReP by Harvest Technologies and the PCCS by Implant Innovations emerge as the most effective and practical devices for office, outpatient surgery center, and wound care center treatment.

References

1. Tozum TF, Demiralp B. Platelet-rich plasma: A promising innovation in dentistry. J Can Dent Assoc 2003;69:664.
2. Carlson NE, Roach RB Jr. Platelet-rich plasma: Clinical applications in dentistry. J Am Dent Assoc 2002;133:1383–1386.
3. John V, Gossweiler M. Implant treatment and the role of platelet-rich plasma. J Indiana Dent Assoc 2003;82(2):8–13.
4. Adler SC, Kent KJ. Enhancing healing with growth factors. Facial Plast Surg Clin North Am 2002;10:129–146.
5. Man D, Plosker H, Winland-Brown JE, Saltz R. The use of autologous platelet-rich plasma (platelet gel) and autologous platelet-poor plasma (fibrin glue) in cosmetic surgery. Plast Reconstr Surg 2001;107:229–237.
6. Crovetti G, Martinelli G, Issi M, et al. Platelet gel for healing cutaneous chronic wounds. Transfus Apheresis Sci 2004;30:145–151.
7. Liu Y, Kalen A, Risto O, Wahlstrom O. Fibroblast proliferation due to exposure to a platelet concentrate in vitro in pH dependent. Wound Repair Regen 2002;10:336–340.
8. Anitua E. The use of plasma-rich growth factors (PRGF) in oral surgery. Pract Proced Aesthet Dent 2001;13:487–493.
9. Kevy S, Jacobson M. Preparation of growth factor enriched autologous platelet gel. Presented at the SVG Biomaterials 27th Annual Meeting, Minneapolis, MN, April 2001.
10. Kassolis JD, Rosen PS, Reynolds MA. Alveolar ridge and sinus augmentation utilizing platelet-rich plasma in combination with freeze-dried bone allograft. Case series. J Periodontol 2000;71:1654-1661.
11. Marx RE. Platelet-rich plasma: Evidence to support its use. J Oral Maxillofac Surg 2004; 62:489–496.
12. Christie RJ, Carrington L, Alving B. Postoperative bleeding induced by topical bovine thrombin: Report of two cases. Surgery 1997;121:708–710.

13. Zehnder JL, Leung LLK. Development of antibodies to thrombin and factor V with recurrent bleeding in a patient exposed to topical bovine thrombin. Blood 1990;76:2011–2016.

14. Rapaport SI, Zivelin A, Minow RA, Hunter CS, Donnelly K. Clinical significance of antibodies to bovine and human thrombin and factor V after surgical use of bovine thrombin. Am J Clin Pathol 1992; 97:84–91.

15. Nichols WL, Daniels TM, Fisher PK, et al. Antibodies to bovine thrombin and coagulation factor V associated with surgical use of topical bovine thrombin or fibrin glue: A frequent finding [abstract]. Blood 1993;82:59.

16. Haynesworth SE, Kodiyala SM, Lang LN, Thomas T, Bruder SP. Mitogenic stimulation of human mesenchymal stem cells by platelet releaseate suggests a mechanism for enhancement of bone repair by platelet concentrates. The 48th Meeting of the Orthopedic Research Society, Dallas, TX, March 2002.

DENTAL APPLICATIONS OF PLATELET-RICH PLASMA

chapter three

Acceleration of Bone Regeneration in Dental Procedures

Bone healing and bone grafting both depend on regeneration of new bone by the mechanisms of cellular proliferation and osteoid synthesis (osteogenesis), on migration of cells into a defect or graft volume (osteoconduction), and on resorption and remodeling into mature bone capable of function (osteoinduction). As related in chapter 1, the involvement of growth factors is inherent in osteogenesis and may be enhanced by elevating the levels of growth factors with platelet-rich plasma (PRP). It is also known that osteoconduction requires the three cell adhesion molecules that are contained within PRP and is enhanced by their increased concentration in the graft. Whether for native bone regeneration or grafting with autogenous bone, allogeneic materials, bone substitutes, or composite grafts, PRP accelerates and enhances the formation of new bone. This chapter describes and demonstrates the direct clinical applications of PRP in the classic sinus lift graft, ridge augmentations, socket preservations, periodontal defects, third molar sockets, and immediate implant placement.

Sinus Lift Grafting

Sinus lift surgery is a relatively new procedure that was developed in the mid-1980s when dental implants became a treatment option in the maxilla. Its singular purpose is to provide sufficient bone in the maxilla to support an implant. The goal of this procedure is to create at least 8 mm and as much as 18 mm of

Table 3-1	Guidelines for Autogenous Bone Requirements and Indications for Use of PRP in Various Patient Types*		
Patient type		Percent autogenous bone required	PRP indicated?
Type Ia Age less than 40 years, no systemic or local tissue compromise		0 to 20	No
Type Ib Age less than 40 years, presence of either a systemic or a local tissue compromise		20 to 50	No
Type Ic Age less than 40 years, presence of both a systemic and a local tissue compromise		20 to 50	Yes
Type IIa Age 40 to 60 years, no systemic or local tissue compromise		20 to 50	No
Type IIb Age 40 to 60 years, presence of either a systemic or a local tissue compromise		20 to 50	Yes
Type IIc Age 40 to 60 years, presence of both a systemic and a local tissue compromise		50 to 80	Yes
Type IIIa Age 60 to 75 years, no systemic or local tissue compromise		50 to 80	Yes
Type IIIb Age 60 to 75 years, presence of either a systemic or a local tissue compromise		50 to 80	Yes
Type IIIc Age 60 to 75 years, presence of both a systemic and a local tissue compromise		80 to 100	Yes
Type IV All individuals 75 years and older		80 to 100	Yes

*Developed by the University of Miami Division of Oral and Maxillofacial Surgery.

implantable bone from the alveolar crest to the newly elevated sinus floor. For this procedure, autogenous bone is the undisputed "gold standard," capable of producing a trabecular bone density of 40% to 60%[1] depending on a variety of factors (eg, the patient's age, systemic health, local tissue quality, and negative influences on healing such as smoking, certain medications, and sinus disease). As noted in chapter 1, PRP plays an important role in accelerating bone regeneration, but it can also blunt the negative influences of age, compromised systemic health, and poor local tissue quality.

While it is true that autogenous bone is the optimal choice of graft material for this procedure, many patients are not candidates for autogenous bone harvesting. Moreover, many practitioners are not trained in extraoral bone harvesting techniques, which are often necessary to graft an entire sinus floor with 100% autogenous bone. Therefore, freeze-dried allogeneic bone,[2] demineralized freeze-dried allogeneic bone,[3] anorganic bovine bone products (eg, Bio-Oss [Osteohealth], PepGen-P15 [Dentsply Friadent CeraMed]),[4] hydroxyapatite products (C-Graft [The Clinician's Preference],[5] Interpore 2000 [Interpore][6]) and other types of bone substitutes are commonly used with reported good results. However, the trabecular bone density of such grafts is much lower than that of autogenous bone,[7,8] varying between 15% and 30%, and the actual clinical outcomes associated with larger sinus lift surgeries, older patients, a local tissue compromise, or a systemic health compromise are often much lower as a result. Therefore, whenever a bone substitute is used in place of autogenous bone and the patient and/or the local tissues are compromised, greater consideration should be given to the use of PRP. Based on broad experience in performing sinus lift grafts in patients of advanced age or affected by osteoporosis, compromised local tissues, and compromised systemic health, the faculty at the University of Miami Division of Oral and Maxillofacial Surgery has developed a set of guidelines (Table 3-1) for combining the use of autogenous bone with bone substitutes and the relative indications for PRP.

Anatomy of the maxillary sinus

The average maxillary sinus volume in the dentate individual is 15 mL compared with an average volume of 21 mL in the edentulous individual, for whom sinus lift grafts are mostly indicated. Since the sinus lift graft will occupy one third of the volume within the floor of the anatomic sinus, about 7 mL of graft material is needed. The sinus extends from the maxillary tuberosity to the interproximal bone between the two maxillary premolar teeth and from the alveolar bone to the undersurface of the orbital floor (Fig 3-1). The maxillary ostium is located at the posterosuperior medial aspect of the sinus (Fig 3-2); because of its location, it depends on the cilia of the sinus membrane to rhythmically advance debris, mucus, and other secretions for drainage (Fig 3-3). In other words, the drainage of a maxillary sinus is not gravity dependent, but relies solely on the health and uncompromised function of the sinus membrane. This unique physiologic feature of the maxillary sinus is of major significance to the sinus lift graft. Sinus membrane friability, edema, and fluid collection have a significant negative effect on the outcome of a sinus lift graft procedure. Such problems occur in association with allergies, viral upper respiratory infections, chronic sinusitis, or previous sinus surgeries. Therefore, an individual with a history of any of these or a panoramic radiograph showing a soft tissue density in a sinus are strongly advised to undergo screening via a computerized tomography (CT) scan (Figs 3-4a and 3-4b). Other individuals do not necessarily require such a screening as part of the preoperative evaluation.

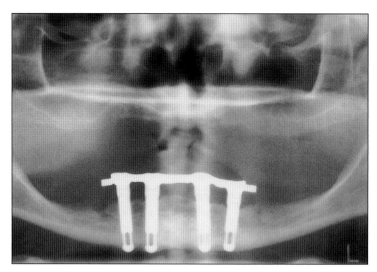

Fig 3-1 The maxillary sinus volume averages 21 mL in the edentulous individual. It extends from the maxillary tuberosity to the first or second premolar area and from the hyperpneumatized alveolar crest to the orbital floor.

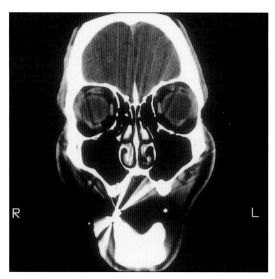

Fig 3-2 The maxillary ostium communicates into the middle meatus of the nose, indicating that sinus drainage is not gravity dependent but requires the action of the ciliated epithelium of the sinus membrane.

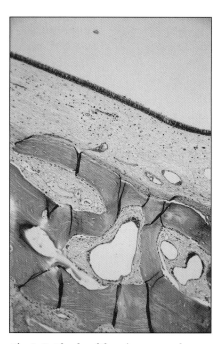

Fig 3-3 The healthy sinus membrane is about 0.30 mm in thickness and has a single layer of pseudostratified columnar epithelium and a loose vascular connective tissue.

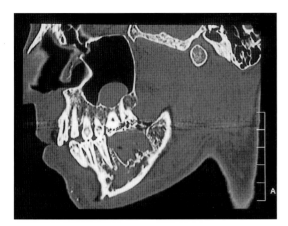

Fig 3-4a The well-known sinus mucocele is a radiographically identifiable condition that represents an inflammation that will negatively affect a sinus lift graft.

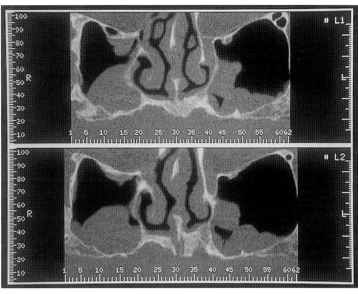

Fig 3-4b If a screening CT scan shows thickened sinus membranes, sinus lift grafting is best deferred in favor of treating the sinus inflammation, or an onlay grafting technique should be used instead.

Patient selection

Although sinus perforation is a common concern of surgeons who perform sinus lift grafting, the perforation of a normal sinus membrane is not associated with loss or failure of the graft (Fig 3-5). Instead, the most common cause of graft loss and/or failure of bone regeneration is sinus inflammation. An otherwise normal, noninflamed sinus perforation will heal within 3 days as a result of the abundant vascularity in the connective tissue wall of the membrane and the single-cell nature of the epithelial lining (see Fig 3-3). However, perforations in edematous and inflamed sinus membranes occur much more readily and do not heal. Moreover, when the graft is then exposed to the toxic environment of the diseased sinus, vascular ingrowth is prohibited. Even if a sinus membrane with chronic inflammation is not perforated, the inflammatory cytokines and digestive enzymes from the inflammation will prevent bone regeneration and consequently resorb the graft. No surgical technique, antibiotic, or growth factor or even PRP can overcome the hostile environment of an inflamed sinus membrane. In such patients, referral to an otorhinolaryngologist and/or treatment leading to a normal CT scan is necessary before a sinus lift graft can be undertaken. If the chronic sinus condition cannot be resolved, alternative approaches that do not require entrance into the sinus environment, such as vertical and/or horizontal ridge augmentation, are recommended.

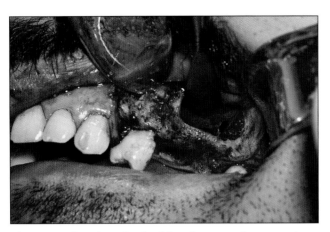

Fig 3-5 Perforation of a healthy sinus membrane such as this is not associated with loss or failure of the graft.

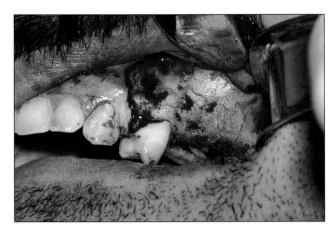

Fig 3-6 A well-extended broad-based flap with a releasing incision is required to adequately access the lateral sinus wall for a sinus lift surgery.

Surgical technique

When performing a sinus lift graft, the surgeon should thoroughly reflect the sinus membrane and place a sufficient quantity of graft material to accommodate the widest and longest implants needed for the reconstruction plan. This will obviate the need for re-grafting later. To support the surgery, complete local anesthetic blocks with or without intravenous sedation are necessary. The full-thickness mucoperiosteal flap used to expose the lateral sinus wall should be broad based and should extend from the maxillary tuberosity to the canine fossa area, where a releasing incision is made (Fig 3-6). The flap should be reflected sufficiently to access the lateral wall of the sinus and therefore should extend superiorly to the infraorbital foramen. Direct visualization of the infraorbital foramen is necessary because it indicates an adequately reflected flap and allows for unrestricted access to the sinus without the danger of tearing or damaging the flap. It also prevents an inadvertent crush injury to the nerve from a retractor placed on the foramen when it cannot be seen.

Entry is made to the sinus in the form of an oval-shaped "window" through the lateral wall and can be accomplished in a couple of ways. The authors prefer to use a large oval finishing bur or diamond bur to paint away the cortical bone (Fig 3-7a). Other surgeons may prefer to use smaller burs to outline an oval bone island, which is then infractured (Fig 3-7b). In either approach, the oval window should be large enough to reflect the sinus membrane directly. For a sinus lift graft in a completely edentulous patient, the authors recommend that the window be 1.5 cm in the inferosuperior dimension and 2.5 cm in the anteroposterior dimension (see Figs 3-7a and 3-7b). At least 3 mm of the lateral wall, between the maxillary crest and the inferior edge of the window, should remain intact.

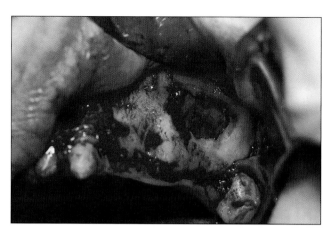 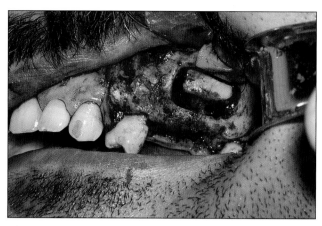

Fig 3-7a The authors recommend a large oval window, 1.5 × 2.5 cm, accomplished by bur reduction of the lateral sinus wall and reflection of the sinus membrane.

Fig 3-7b Alternatively, an oval window of the same size can be created by means of the infracture technique, which leaves a lateral cortical segment attached to the sinus membrane.

Reflection of the sinus membrane should ideally begin at the sinus floor. After mobilizing a small amount of sinus membrane in this area, however, the membrane elevators should encircle the oval opening, releasing the sinus membrane circumferentially around the opening. The surgeon should then return to the sinus floor area to reflect additional membrane. This method will minimize tears to the membrane by releasing areas of adherence around the superior, anterior, and posterior edges of the oval opening. The sinus membrane should then be thoroughly elevated. The surgeon should reflect the membrane posteriorly as far as the tuberosity and across the entire floor of the sinus to reach the medial wall. Failure to reflect the sinus membrane from the medial wall is a common mistake in sinus lift grafts that will lead to medial notching of the graft and in turn may limit the length of implant that can be accommodated (Fig 3-8).

Once the sinus membrane is completely elevated, the authors recommend soaking a cottonoid packing (Codman Surgical Patties, Johnson & Johnson) in either a local anesthetic solution with 1:100,000 epinephrine or in 4% cocaine solution and placing it into the sinus lift cavity for 3 to 5 minutes (Fig 3-9a). This packing will allow the area to achieve absolute hemostasis and will reflect the sinus membrane a bit further. More importantly, it will give the surgeon a more direct and unobscured view of the sinus that will allow a more complete membrane reflection and therefore the placement of a greater amount of graft material (Figs 3-9b and 3-9c).

Even the most skilled surgeons will experience sinus membrane perforations; estimates of the incidence range from 10% to 40%, and the average is somewhere around 25%.[9] As noted earlier, a healthy sinus membrane can heal and reseal the sinus air space from the graft, and PRP can accelerate this process. If the perforation is small (less than 2 mm), it can be covered with a PRP membrane

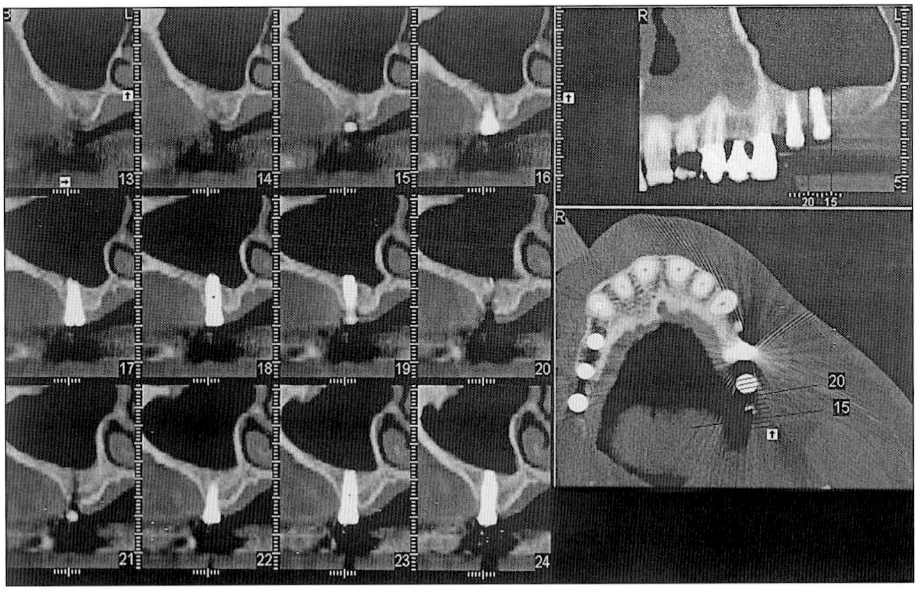

Fig 3-8 An incompletely reflected sinus membrane will result in a size- and volume-deficient graft and compromised implant placement.

(Fig 3-10), which is made by activating 1.0 to 1.5 mL of PRP on a smooth surface for 1 minute to allow a mature clot to form. The fibrin network of the PRP clot will act as a scaffold for membrane healing, and the growth factors in PRP will accelerate the healing process. If the perforation is of medium size (between 2 and 10 mm), a collagen membrane reconstituted with activated PRP will be more effective (Fig 3-11). The added structure of the collagen membrane will prevent particles of graft material from passing through the larger perforation, and the PRP within it will accelerate migration of the sinus membrane over the framework of the collagen membrane. If the perforation is large (greater than 10 mm), a crosslinked collagen membrane (such as BioMend Extend [Zimmer Dental] or Bio-Gide [Geistlich Biomaterials]) together with activated PRP is recommended (Fig 3-12). Because it is more firmly structured and has a delayed absorption, this type of membrane will also prevent the particulate graft material from extruding through this larger perforation while acting as a scaffold for the PRP-accelerated sinus membrane migration.

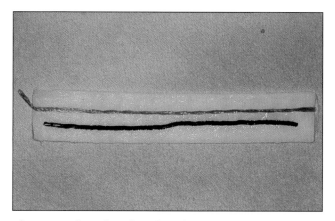

Fig 3-9a After elevating the sinus membrane, a 0.5 × 3–inch surgical pad (cottonoid) soaked in a local anesthetic solution with 1:100,000 epinephrine can be packed into the prepared sinus lift cavity. This will achieve hemostasis, gain additional membrane reflection, and allow assessment of the graft volume.

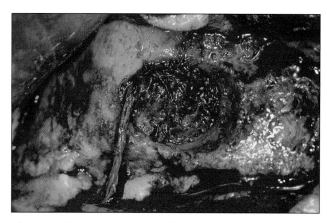

Fig 3-9b The cottonoid is gently packed into place and left for at least 5 minutes before removal.

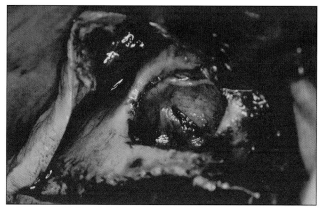

Fig 3-9c Once the pad is removed, hemostasis is evident. The technique can be repeated several times if necessary.

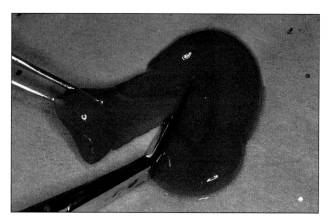

Fig 3-10 A PRP membrane is created when a small pool of PRP placed in a container is allowed to clot. The membrane can then be cut to the appropriate dimensions and placed over a small sinus perforation as a biologic patch.

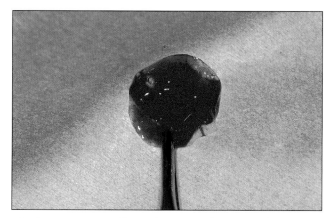

Fig 3-11 For a medium sinus membrane perforation, a CollaTape membrane (Zimmer Dental) can be saturated with PRP and used as a patch. Alternatively, a dry piece of CollaTape can be placed over the perforation site and then saturated with PRP.

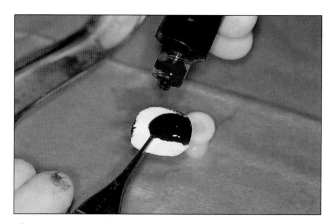

Fig 3-12 BioMend, a long-lasting, relatively rigid collagen membrane, can be used for large tears. The membrane can be saturated prior to sinus placement or placed dry and then saturated with PRP.

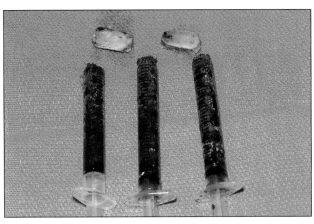 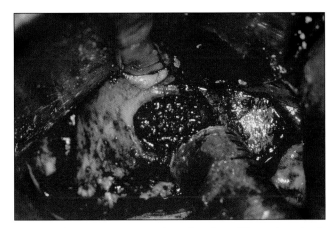

Figs 3-13a and 3-13b A 3-mL syringe can be used to "inject" a compacted autogenous graft into the sinus lift cavity, which is then upregulated with PRP.

Placement of the sinus lift graft

Using 100% autogenous bone

It is important to remember that the amount of bone regenerated from an autogenous bone graft depends on the number of endosteal osteoblasts and marrow stem cells that are transplanted. These numbers may be increased both mechanically, by packing the graft material densely into the defect, and biochemically, by exposing them to the mitogenic growth factors in PRP. Autogenous cancellous marrow grafts can be optimized mechanically by placing portions of the graft sequentially into a 3-mL syringe from the removed plunger end and compacted by activating the plunger. Once the barrel is filled, the tip of the syringe is cut off so that the compacted graft can be expressed into the reflected sinus lift cavity (Figs 3-13a and 3-13b). The graft may be further compacted within the sinus lift surgical site using amalgam pluggers or bone compactors. Before compacting it at the site, however, the autogenous graft may be incubated with activated PRP. This will allow the secreted growth factors to bind the graft cell membranes, and it will also allow the fibrin, fibronectin, and vitronectin cell adhesion proteins to bind the graft particles together, thereby improving the handling properties of the graft (Fig 3-14a). To be maximally effective, this incubation must proceed for 1 hour in order for the platelets to secrete 90% or more of their pre-synthesized growth factors. Waiting less than 1 hour may cause them to lose some of their effectiveness. Therefore, we recommend that a small volume of PRP should be placed into the sinus cavity first, followed by additional increments of PRP as more graft material is placed. The authors also recommend using some of the PRP as a covering for the graft once it is placed (Fig 3-14b). In this fashion, the growth factors will contact the overlying mucosa and also trickle down through the graft. This will accelerate soft tissue healing, thereby reducing wound dehiscences and graft exposures. The result is a rapid regeneration of bone in the sinus with sufficient height and width to accommodate longer and wider dental implants (Fig 3-14c).

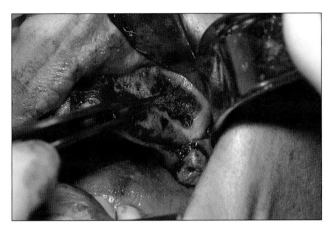

Fig 3-14a Particulate grafts incubated in activated PRP gain adherence and may be introduced into the sinus lift cavity with forceps and compressed once in place.

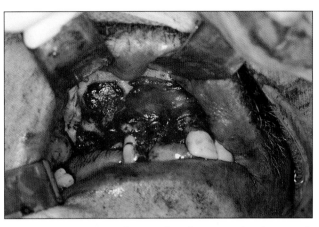

Fig 3-14b A PRP membrane placed over an implant graft and sinus lift window will provide growth factors and cell adhesion molecules both to the graft and to the overlying mucosal flap.

Fig 3-14c A well-reflected sinus membrane, an autogenous bone graft, and PRP result in rapid bone regeneration and significant volume of bone for placement of the dental implant.

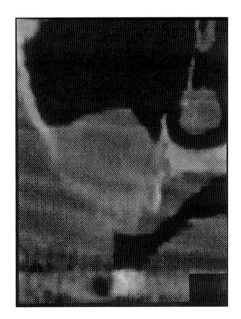

Using 100% allogeneic bone

Allogeneic bone contains so little bone morphogenetic protein (BMP) (2.5×10^{-6} µg/mg of allogeneic bone) as to be essentially noninductive. When 100% allogeneic bone is used in a sinus lift graft, bone regeneration occurs only via osteoconduction, whereby endosteal osteoblasts and marrow mesenchymal stem cells from the bony walls of the sinus and to a lesser extent from the sinus membrane migrate into the sinus cavity to deposit viable bone onto the nonviable allogeneic bone. Therefore, when allogeneic bone is used, it is advisable to place activated PRP into the prepared sinus surgical site first and to incubate the graft material with activated PRP before placing it into the site (Fig 3-15). This allows the growth factors in PRP to act on the endosteal osteoblasts and marrow stem cells

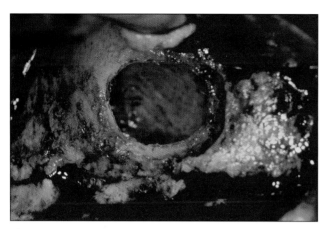

Fig 3-15 Once the sinus membrane is adequately reflected, a small amount of PRP should be sprayed into the site to coat the membrane prior to placement of allogeneic graft materials.

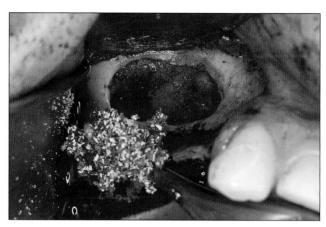

Fig 3-16 Allogeneic bone particles are easier to place with the adherence gained from the cell adhesion molecules in PRP.

of the bony sinus walls, while the fibrin, fibronectin, and vitronectin adhere collectively to the allogeneic bone particles. The result is enhanced cellular migration and regenerative bone deposition on the allogeneic bone. In addition, the clotted nature of PRP will improve the handling properties of the allogeneic bone particles and make them easier to place (Fig 3-16). It is important to remember that osteoconduction of bone works by signaling growth factors and requires a scaffold for osteoprogenitor cell migration. PRP provides both of these. In fact, the regenerative bone deposited on the surface of the allogeneic bone is promoted by PRP and migrates along the allogeneic bone surface upon the fibrin strands adhering to the surface (see chapter 1, Figs 1-37a to 1-37d).

Using bone substitutes

PRP enhances regeneration of new bone around grafts made of bone substitutes by a mechanism similar to that of allogeneic bone. Therefore, the authors again recommend placing activated PRP into the prepared sinus lift surgical site and incubating the graft material in activated PRP. However, with bone substitutes, it is important not only to incubate the material in PRP, but also to develop the material into a well-formed PRP clot (Fig 3-17). The reason is that, despite manufacturers' claims to the contrary, bone substitutes do not have the same surface characteristics or pore size as bone. Therefore, bone substitutes rely more on fibrin's adherence to their surface to promote osteoconduction of regenerative bone from the adjacent sinus walls. Incorporating the bone substitute particles into the PRP maximizes the number of cell adhesion molecules on their surface and at the same time prevents them from becoming too densely packed. Unlike autogenous bone, bone substitutes should not be mechanically compacted. To do so reduces the interparticle space, which inhibits sufficient vascular in-growth and thus results in the formation of fibrous tissue rather than bone.

Fig 3-17 Most bone substitutes are small particles that gain improved handling properties when activated PRP is applied.

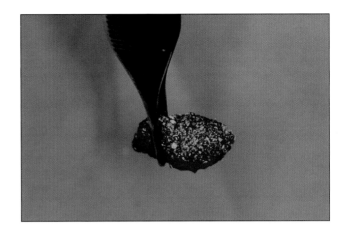

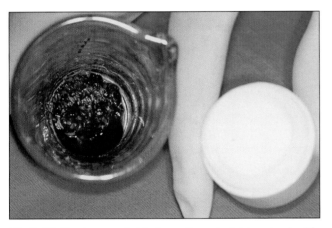

Fig 3-18 The bone substitute graft material is mixed with activated PRP prior to being placed into the maxillary sinus.

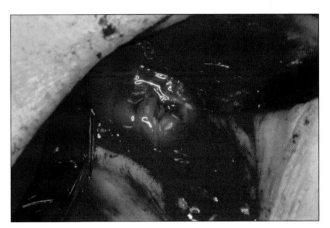

Fig 3-19 A PRP membrane can be used to cover the oval opening of the lateral sinus wall.

Using composites of autogenous bone and bone substitutes/allogeneic bone

When autogenous bone is combined with bone substitutes, the aim is to transplant both endosteal osteoblasts and marrow stem cells from the autogenous bone and use the bone substitute/allogeneic bone to provide a matrix. Therefore, the formation of regenerative bone in the sinus lift will result in part from graft osteogenesis and in part from osteoconduction from the surrounding bone. In this scenario, the autogenous graft and bone substitute or allogeneic bone is mixed together and incorporated as a composite into the PRP clot (Fig 3-18). This composite is then placed into the prepared sinus lift cavity, and a PRP membrane is placed over the oval opening of the lateral sinus wall (Fig 3-19).

Ridge Augmentation Grafting

Augmenting a maxillary or mandibular ridge to accommodate dental implants may take the form of horizontal ridge augmentation, vertical ridge augmentation, or simultaneous horizontal-vertical ridge augmentation. In all of these, protecting the graft from masticatory and/or provisional denture forces is necessary throughout the period of revascularization and cell proliferation whether PRP is used or not. If PRP is used, the graft will need to be protected for 3 weeks; if PRP is not used, it may be vulnerable for up to 6 weeks.[1,10] To protect the graft, the surgeon may need to prohibit the patient from wearing a provisional appliance, affix the appliance so that it does not compress the graft, relieve the undersurface of the provisional appliance, immobilize the jaws, or adjust the occlusion as necessary.

Horizontal ridge augmentation

Horizontal ridge augmentation can be accomplished following one of two basic approaches. Where possible, a ridge may be split using a bur and ridge-splitting osteotomes and an implant immediately placed between the redefined buccal and lingual cortices along with an interpositional graft material of the surgeon's choice. PRP is used between the split cortices and within the graft material in such cases, and in addition it may be necessary to cover the split ridge with a membrane to restrict fibrous growth into the split ridge. A PRP membrane may be used in place of and without a commercial membrane since it provides the advantages of growth factor enhancement to both the soft tissue flap and the bony ridge.

When an extreme knife-edge ridge configuration or inelastic cortices prohibit ridge-splitting, onlay grafting is used. Depending on the size and shape required, onlay grafts may be harvested from the ramus, chin, calvaria, or anterior/posterior ilium. Because onlay grafts undergo significant resorption-remodeling, the volume of the graft is reduced by as much as 25% to 40% within 6 months of placement. Calvarial bone undergoes the smallest reduction in volume (15% to 25% over 6 months) because it revascularizes more quickly than other graft sources by virtue of its abundant Volkmann and Haversian canals, which are part of its natural diploic vascular communications to the brain. To minimize graft reduction, absolute graft immobility, supplementation with compacted cancellous marrow, and PRP should be used. Graft immobilization can be achieved with lag-screws, which firmly compress the onlay graft to the host bone surface (Fig 3-20). To use the lag screw most effectively, a single bur hole is drilled through the graft and into the host bone. The bur hole is then overdrilled in the graft to a diameter slightly larger than the diameter of the screw. This will produce a true lag-screw compression. Two screws must be placed into each onlay graft to prevent rotation around a single screw (see Fig 3-20). Before the graft is secured to the host bone, activated PRP should be placed in the contact area between them to accelerate and enhance their union. Once the onlay grafts are in place, compacted cancellous marrow should ideally be placed and compacted around these block grafts and also placed into any voids or crevices created by the graft contours (Fig 3-21). Several layers of PRP should then be placed over this block onlay graft

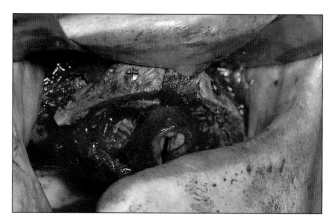

Fig 3-20 Autogenous corticocancellous grafts lag-screwed to the lateral maxilla as part of a horizontal ridge augmentation surgery.

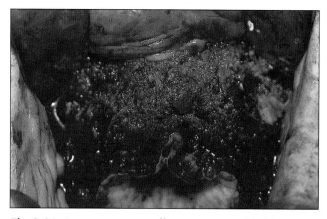

Fig 3-21 Autogenous cancellous marrow added between and on the surface of corticocancellous blocks lag-screwed to the maxilla.

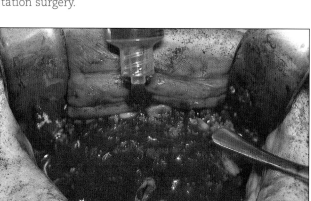

Fig 3-22a Layer of activated PRP added over the surface of the grafts.

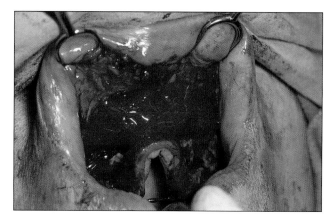

Fig 3-22b Activated PRP maturing on the graft surface.

Fig 3-23 Collagen membrane over the graft-PRP complex.

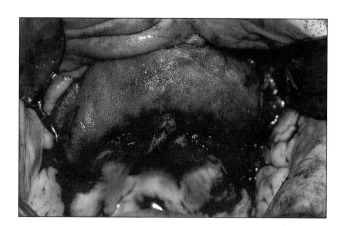

and cancellous marrow composite to incorporate them together and maximize the advantages of PRP's growth factors and cell adhesion molecules (Figs 3-22a and 3-22b). Due to the scarred nature of the periosteum, it will have lost its osteogenic nature and thus will contribute only fibrous growth into the graft. Therefore the surgeon should consider placing a membrane over this graft composite (Fig 3-23). Adding PRP to the membrane surface will minimize the potential for flap

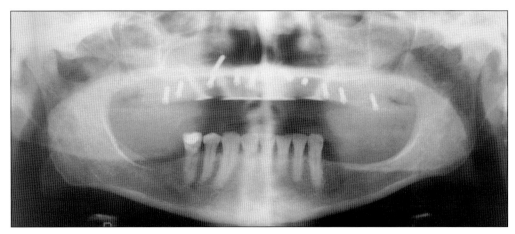

Fig 3-24a Panoramic radiograph of the horizontal ridge augmentation graft shown in Figs 3-20 to 3-23. Good bone graft placement and consolidation are evident.

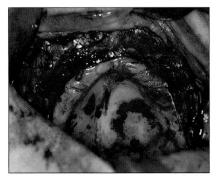

Fig 3-24b Re-entry at 3 months shows mature graft before removal of screws.

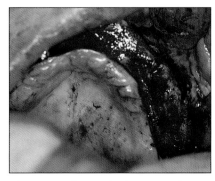

Fig 3-24c The graft shows good contour and bone density for implant placement.

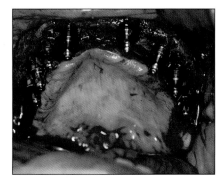

Fig 3-24d Grafts that regenerate a dense bone with good arch form and bone volume allow for ideal implant positioning.

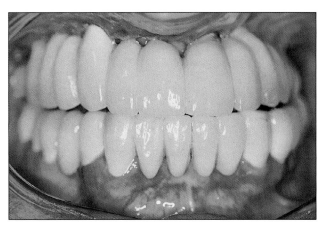

Fig 3-24e Cemented fixed restoration after maxillary complete-arch horizontal ridge augmentation.

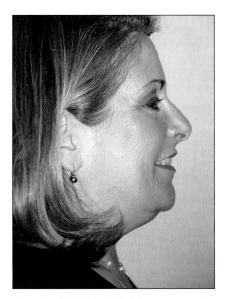

Fig 3-24f Horizontal ridge augmentation of the maxilla provides upper lip support and esthetic balance of the nose-lip-chin profile.

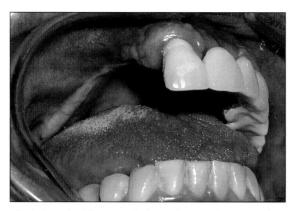

Fig 3-25 Significant soft tissue loss and contraction often accompany a vertical bone deficiency.

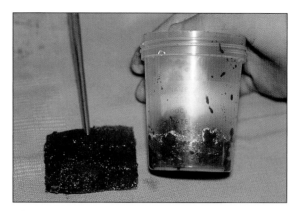

Fig 3-26 Vertical ridge augmentation often requires a larger graft than that needed for horizontal ridge augmentation; therefore, larger autogenous blocks from the ilium, additional cancellous marrow, and PRP are often needed.

dehiscence and membrane exposure. Horizontal ridge augmentation enhanced with PRP is suitable for implant placement 3 months after grafting (Figs 3-24a to 3-24f).

Vertical ridge augmentation

Vertical ridge augmentation is more difficult than horizontal ridge augmentation due to the restriction of the soft tissues, usually from scar contractions (Fig 3-25), and the greater practical difficulty of protecting the graft from masticatory forces. In some cases, sufficient bone remains so that an osteotomy may be accomplished and the segment distracted vertically. Too often, however, there is insufficient natural bone stock to accomplish distraction, or the defect will not accommodate a commercial distractor, leaving onlay bone grafting as the only option available. Like horizontal ridge augmentation, vertical ridge augmentation is most successful using autogenous bone harvested as a corticocancellous block from the ramus, chin, calvarium, or anterior/posterior ilium (Fig 3-26). These block grafts follow the same pattern of resorption/remodeling encountered in horizontal bone grafts. As an alternative, with vertical ridge augmentation it is possible to use an all-cancellous marrow graft placed in a titanium basket crib for larger defects or under a titanium-reinforced membrane for smaller defects. If onlay grafts are used to gain vertical height in the maxilla or mandible, the use of rigid lag-screw fixation (Fig 3-27a), supplementation with additional cancellous marrow (Fig 3-27b), application of PRP (Fig 3-27c), and membrane coverage are as important to this procedure as they are to horizontal ridge augmentation. Of added importance in vertical ridge augmentation is the need for soft tissue undermining and advancement over the graft to gain an absolutely tension-free closure; merely scoring the periosteum is not sufficient. The undermining must be thorough, carrying well into the labial or the buccal mucosa, and at a very superficial level in order to

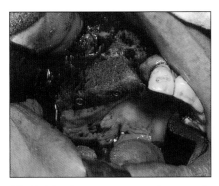

Fig 3-27a Autogenous corticocancellous graft lag-screwed to the deficient maxilla.

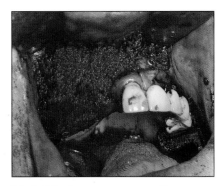

Fig 3-27b Autogenous cancellous marrow added to the corticocancellous graft.

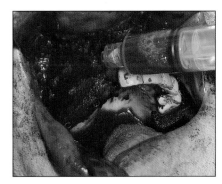

Fig 3-27c PRP added on top of the autogenous corticocancellous block–cancellous marrow composite.

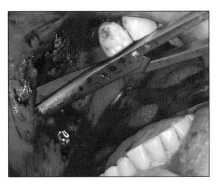

Fig 3-27d To cover the added contours created by a vertical augmentation graft, the mucosa must be significantly undermined at a superficial level so as to separate the mucosa from its muscle attachments and allow for flap advancement.

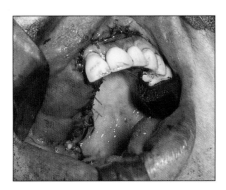

Fig 3-27e The undermined flap is advanced for a tension-free closure over the graft.

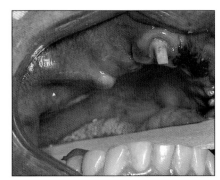

Fig 3-27f A corticocancellous block will remodel, losing about 0.5 mm of height per month. Tension of the mucosa from the screw heads is a result of graft remodeling and mucosal contraction.

separate any muscle attachments to the flap (Fig 3-27d). Remaining muscle activity in the flap will promote microscopic salivary leakage and allow bacterial ingress through the closure by its pulling action on the flap. This can cause a subtle infection and lead to failure of bone regeneration by the graft or dehiscence resulting in graft exposure. The flap must be advanced sufficiently to achieve an everted edge-to-edge closure with laxity (Fig 3-27e). Due to the critical importance of healing without dehiscence, placing PRP on the flap edges as well as over the surface of the bone graft at the time of closure is recommended. The result will be a mature graft with a bone height similar to that of the adjacent alveolar cleft. Therefore, dental implants can be placed with their emergence profiles at the alveolar cleft (Figs 3-27f to 3-27i). This will allow for fixed (cemented) restorations with a level occlusal plane and a more natural appearance (Figs 3-27j and 3-27k).

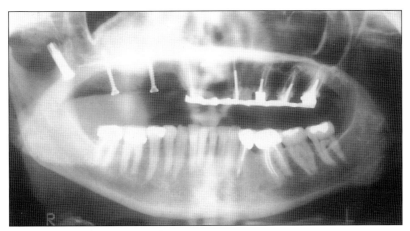

Fig 3-27g Panoramic radiograph of a vertical augmentation graft affixed with fixation screws. A dental implant has also been placed into the pterygoid plates to support a provisional prosthesis that will avoid placing compressive forces on the graft.

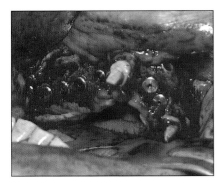

Fig 3-27h After 4 months the graft is mature and dense enough for implant placement.

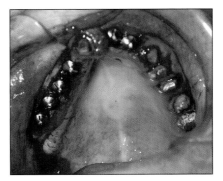

Fig 3-27i The augmentation should achieve near-ideal arch form and height so that the implants will match the cementoenamel junction of the native teeth and blend into a natural-appearing contour.

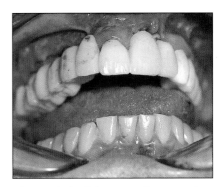

Fig 3-27j Fixed (cemented) restoration made possible by complete regeneration of alveolar height and arch form.

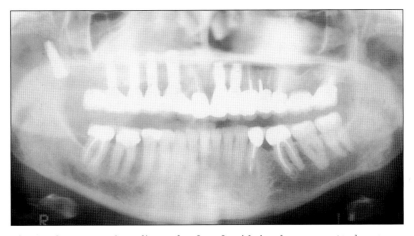

Fig 3-27k Panoramic radiograph of graft with implant-supported restorations. Graft height is comparable to that of native bone.

71

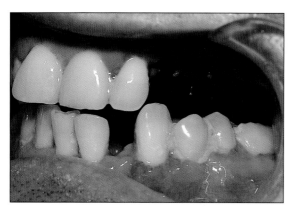

Fig 3-28a Traumatic alveolar vertical bone loss associated with fracture of the mandible.

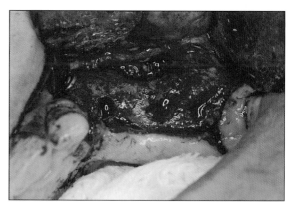

Fig 3-28b Traumatic vertical and horizontal ridge deficiency.

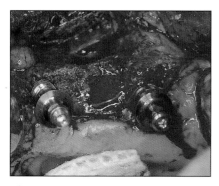

Fig 3-28c Implants seated into native bone with several threads intentionally positioned coronal to the bone to achieve a tenting concept.

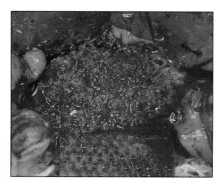

Fig 3-28d Cancellous marrow placed around and to the height of the implants. A 3-month resorbable membrane is positioned with fixation to the palatal bone.

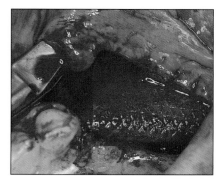

Fig 3-28e Undermining the flap in a superficial plane is necessary to advance the flap and eliminate muscle pull.

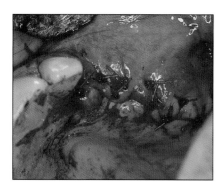

Fig 3-28f Undermined and advanced flap closed without tension over the contour gain of the graft.

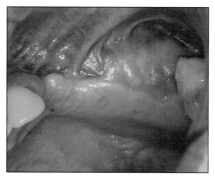

Fig 3-28g Wide ridge and good height gained by the graft allow for a fixed (cemented) restoration.

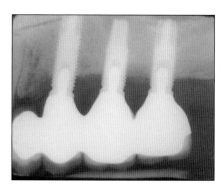

Fig 3-28h Fixed (cemented) partial denture completes the rehabilitation. Note the bone height and density achieved.

If a titanium basket crib or a reinforced membrane is used, a 100% cancellous marrow or cancellous marrow mixed with a maximum of 50% allogeneic bone/bone substitute should be incorporated into PRP within this containment (Figs 3-28a to 3-28d). In addition, layers of PRP should be placed over this graft-basket-membrane composite and along the soft tissue closure to prevent exposure of the titanium basket or the reinforced membrane. The result is bone regeneration within the volume space created by the basket crib or the reinforced membrane. In the case shown in Figs 3-28a and 3-28b, the implants also help to tent the membrane and the mucosa. Therefore, the result can be expected to achieve a bone height equal to that of the adjacent bone and support a fixed (cemented) restoration (Figs 3-28e to 3-28h).

Third Molar Sockets

Despite improvements in surgical technique and the use of intrasocket and even systemic antibiotics, third molar surgery continues to be associated with two well-known complications. The first is alveolar osteitis (commonly known as dry socket), which has a reported incidence ranging from 2% to 18%,[11] with the average individual's risk between 6% and 8%.[12] The second is reduced bone regeneration in the third molar socket, particularly in the area adjacent to the second molar, which often creates a food trap and a pathologic periodontal pocket. Separate studies by Babbush[13] and by Mancuso et al[14] have demonstrated the remarkable ability of PRP both to reduce the incidence of dry socket and to enhance bone regeneration in the socket, thereby reducing patients' risks of developing infrabony periodontal pockets and a pathologic condition at the distal aspect of the second molar.

Alveolar osteitis is primarily a bacterial digestion of the blood clot and a colonization of the bony surface, which provokes inflammation and results in reduced bone regeneration in a third molar socket. The inflammation explains the painful nature of alveolar osteitis, and the bacterial colonization and degradation of the blood clot itself explains the foul odor and taste associated with this condition. What separates an alveolar osteitis from a true osteomyelitis is only the fact that these bacteria do not invade the marrow space of the mandible. In rare instances, however, alveolar osteitis will progress to the more serious condition of osteomyelitis.

When alveolar osteitis develops, the focus of the patient and the practitioner is on relieving the pain and preventing its progression into an osteomyelitis. Irrigating the socket, packing it with various medicaments, and sometimes using systemic antibiotics almost always relieves the pain and resolves the condition within 1 week. The socket finally develops granulation tissue, and epithelium from the adjacent mucosa migrates over the granulation tissue to cover the socket. Bone slowly regenerates by migrating through the granulation tissue (osteoconduction) from the bony walls of the socket. Nonetheless, a critical analysis of the sockets complicated by alveolar osteitis has revealed a reduced bone height and an absence of bone around the distal root of the second molar, predisposing it to root caries and unresolvable periodontitis (Fig 3-29). The reduced amount of bone is the direct result of loss of the blood clot and of the seven growth factors naturally secreted by the platelets contained within it, as well as loss of the fibrin-fibronectin-vitronectin cell adhesion molecules that normally enhance osteoconduction of the growth factor–stimulated osteoprogenitor cells from the bony walls of the socket. The study by Mancuso et al showed evidence of the significantly reduced clinical symptoms of dry sockets when treated with PRP. This randomized, samepatient controlled, split-mouth study of 117 patients reported a 12.8% incidence of dry socket in the side without PRP versus only 3.4% in the side treated with PRP, representing an almost fourfold decrease. The study also showed a superior final bone height in the PRP-treated socket as compared to the non–PRP-treated site.[14] Babbush's extensive experience using PRP in third molar sockets confirmed the data published by Mancuso et al. Moreover, he has shown elimination of the periodontal defect adjacent to the second molar tooth (Figs 3-30a to 3-30d). Babbush reported the complete elimination of this defect and development of a bone height that was level with the height of the second molar bone following the use of C-Graft, Bio-Oss, or PepGen P-15 combined with PRP.[13]

The mechanism by which PRP prevents alveolar osteitis and leads to enhanced bone regeneration remains uncertain at this time. It may be as simple as PRP's acid pH of 6.5 to 6.7, which is known to inhibit bacterial colony growth. The acid pH in a native blood clot, by comparison, is 7.4. PRP's lower pH is a result of the citric acid (anticoagulant citrate dextrose A [ACD-A]) that is used as an anticoagulant in its development. Another possibility is the fact that PRP concentrates white blood cells as well as platelets. Most PRP research has focused on platelet concentration, their growth factors, and the cell adhesion molecules in PRP, and not on the benefit of concentrating leukocytes. It is possible that a reduction in alveolar osteitis is a clinical manifestation of the bacterial inhibition afforded by the greater numbers of functioning viable leukocytes. A third theory is that PRP's rapid development of granulation tissue with early ingrowth of capillaries prevents bacterial growth by bringing in circulating macrophages and neutrophils and by creating a more oxygen-rich environment that specifically suppresses the growth of anaerobic microorganisms. It is likely that all three of these mechanisms play a role in the action of PRP.

Current evidence does not suggest the need to use PRP in all third molar surgeries at this time; it may be neither practical nor cost effective to do so. However, surgeons should consider PRP use when third molar surgery is planned in an individual at heightened risk for alveolar osteitis, including women taking birth control pills, smokers, individuals with a history of pericoronitis, individuals older than 30 years, patients on steroids or undergoing chemotherapy, patients with a history of previous radiation to the surgical area, type I and type II diabetics, and patients with impacted third molars for which the trauma of surgery is expected to be somewhat greater than usual.

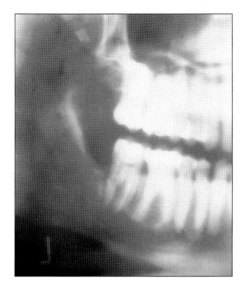

Fig 3-29 Reduced bone regeneration, a periodontal defect, and subsequent root caries resulting from an alveolar osteitis.

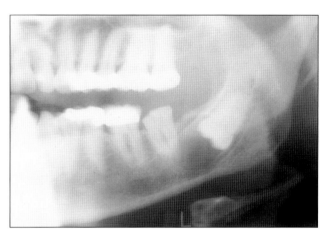

Fig 3-30a Complete bony impaction of third molar with a dentigerous cyst.

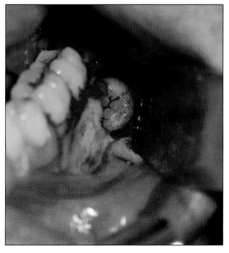

Fig 3-30b Impacted tooth with associated bony defect as shown in Fig 3-30a.

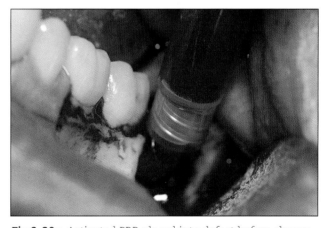

Fig 3-30c Activated PRP placed into defect before closure.

Fig 3-30d One-year postoperative radiograph from surgery depicted in Figs 3-30a to 3-30c shows excellent bone regeneration and bone height.

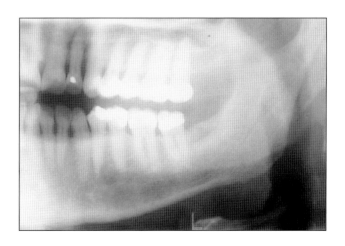

Periodontal Defect Treatment

Periodontal defects form as a result of a disease process that is initiated by the presence of subgingival microorganisms. The toxins from these microorganisms provoke a constant inflammatory state that gradually breaks down the epithelial attachment and leads to resorption of the alveolar bone. Left untreated, periodontal bone loss will progress to tooth mobility and eventually to tooth loss. Indeed, periodontal disease represents the leading cause of tooth loss worldwide. Regenerating bone in periodontal defects has been shown to reduce tooth mobility and prevent tooth loss, but bone regeneration can take place only after the disease process has been arrested.[15] Therefore, before attempting to regenerate bone in these defects, the clinician must thoroughly debride the defect and plane the exposed root surfaces. Next, a graft material and a grafting technique must be selected based on their ability to withstand the hostile environment of a periodontal defect and adapt to the size and anatomic constraints of the bone defect and overlying soft tissues. In this context, treatment of a periodontal defect relies as much on soft tissue wound healing as it does on bone regeneration. Therefore, PRP, which already has an established role and expanding applications in periodontal defect surgery,[16,17] should be seriously considered for use in most cases. Specifically, several authors have shown superior bone regeneration in human intrabony defects when porous bovine bone is combined with PRP as compared with the use of porous bovine bone alone.[18] Similarly, PRP produced improved results when combined with several graft materials as compared with use of the same graft materials without PRP, including calcium sulfate,[19] tricalcium phosphate,[20] allogeneic bone,[21] autogenous bone, and composites of autogenous and allogeneic bone.

The surgical approach to the treatment of a periodontal defect requires a sulcular incision that extends well past the defect site to allow sufficient flap reflection that will enable the surgeon to visualize the entire defect and suture the flap over a well-supported bony base. The granulation tissue in the defect must be thoroughly debrided and the root surfaces planed. The defect may be irrigated with saline or Peridex (Teva) or washed with citric acid and then irrigated with saline to remove any acid residue. Plain or distilled water should not be used as an irrigant because its hypotonicity can disrupt the cell membranes of host or grafted cells and result in reduced bone regeneration.[22] Regardless of the type of graft materials used, PRP will enhance the rate of healing and the degree of bone regeneration. The authors recommend incubating the graft material in PRP while the defect is being debrided and irrigated. By this means, the cell adhesion molecules and the clotting nature of the PRP will bind the graft material into a working composite that will be easier to handle. Once the graft material is placed into the defect, the authors recommend placing a layer of activated PRP over the surface of the graft (Figs 3-31a to 3-31e). In this fashion, the growth factors secreted by the platelets in PRP will directly contact the mucoperiosteal flap used to cover the graft and at the same time trickle down into the graft to accelerate both the soft tissue healing and the bone regeneration.

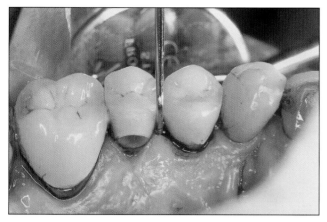

Fig 3-31a A 9-mm periodontal defect as it is being measured with a probe. The canine and the two premolars have lost part of the lingual alveolar bone as a result of periodontitis. (Figs 3-31a to 3-31e courtesy of Dr Jack T. Krauser, Boca Raton, Florida.)

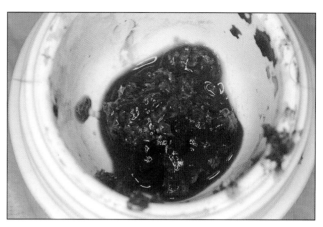

Fig 3-31b Allogeneic graft materials such as Puros (Zimmer Dental) mixed with PRP have proven to be effective in replacing the lost bone in these types of defects. Here the graft material is saturated with PRP.

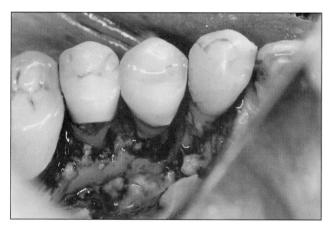

Fig 3-31c Once the flap is reflected, the dimensions of the defect can be fully appreciated.

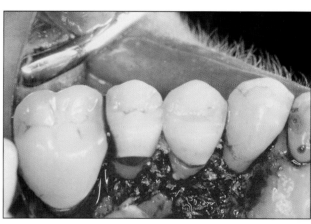

Fig 3-31d In addition to providing growth factors, PRP enhances the handling properties of the graft material as it holds all the bone graft particles together and makes molding it against the defect much easier.

Fig 3-31e Three-week postoperative view showing accelerated healing of the tissues.

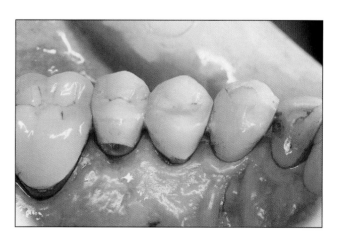

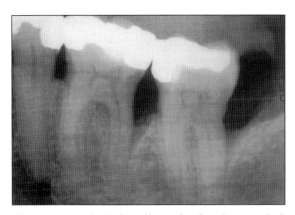

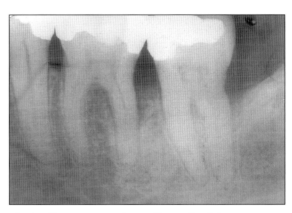

Fig 3-32a Periapical radiograph showing vertical bone loss on the distal surfaces of the roots of two mandibular molars. (Figs 3-32a and 3-32b courtesy of Dr Jack T. Krauser, Boca Raton, Florida.)

Fig 3-32b Postoperative radiograph of the same two mandibular molars where new bone formation can be observed 6 weeks after grafting with allogeneic bone (Puros) together with PRP.

In this application, PRP can be expected to expedite healing of the soft tissue over the graft and thereby reduce the potential for dehiscence and sequestration of graft particles. It can also be expected to hasten bone regeneration in the defect and cause the formation of a more dense bone, even when the graft material contains no autogenous osteoprogenitor cells (Figs 3-32a and 3-32b). These benefits can be attributed to the presence of the PRP-secreted growth factors on the bony walls adjacent to the defect. Specifically, the platelet-derived growth factor (PDGF) and transforming growth factor beta (TGFβ) isomers stimulate proliferation of host endosteal osteoblasts and marrow stem cells; the growth factors TGFβ1 and TGFβ2 prompt differentiation of the marrow stem cells along osteoblastic lines; the vascular endothelial growth factor (VEGF) promotes capillary ingrowth to provide the nutrients and oxygen needed to synthesize osteoid; and the cell adhesion molecules fibrin, fibronectin, and vitronectin coat the nonviable graft particles and root surface and enable development of a matrix that connects the host bony walls to the graft particles and to the root surface. This is the matrix on which osteoid is deposited and the means by which new, microscopically visible bone forms over the surface of the nonviable bone particles. This process of osteoconduction requires cell proliferation, differentiation, and migration, and finally new bone formation, all of which are enhanced by the constituents of PRP (Figs 3-33a to 3-33e).

If autogenous cancellous graft material is used, either alone or in combination with a nonviable graft material, the cell population of the graft will be influenced by the same growth factors and cell adhesion molecules and in the same manner as described for a nonviable graft. However, the endosteal osteoblasts and mesenchymal stem cells transferred into the defect by the autogenous graft will be acted upon to produce osteoid and to speed bone maturation. When autogenous graft material is used, there are even more cells available for upregulation by PRP, and migration is unnecessary since these cells are already positioned within the defect. For these reasons, combining autogenous bone with any other graft material transplants the capacity for osteogenesis into the defect, which already possesses the capacity for osteoconduction via the nonviable graft material. Since one- and two-wall bony defects have a small surface area of native bone and hence a

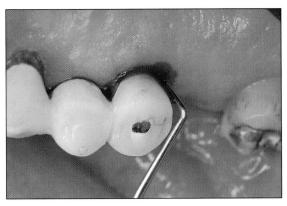

Fig 3-33a Maxillary premolar in a multi-unit fixed partial denture presents a 7-mm-deep pocket. (Figs 3-33a to 3-33e courtesy of Dr Jack T. Krauser, Boca Raton, Florida.)

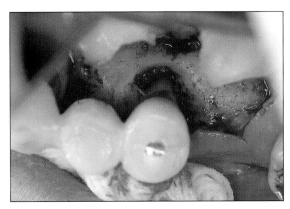

Fig 3-33b Upon flap reflection, the saucer-like defect can be fully appreciated.

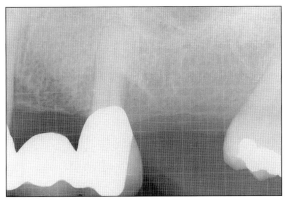

Fig 3-33c Radiographic view reveals that the premolar has lost approximately 50% of its supporting bone.

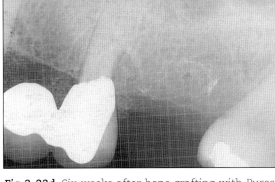

Fig 3-33d Six weeks after bone grafting with Puros and PRP, new bone appears to be properly maturing around the premolar, as demonstrated by the trabecular bone pattern in this radiograph.

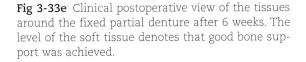

Fig 3-33e Clinical postoperative view of the tissues around the fixed partial denture after 6 weeks. The level of the soft tissue denotes that good bone support was achieved.

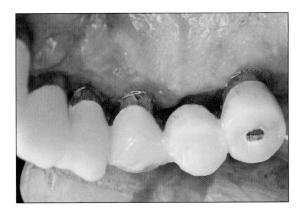

diminished host osteoprogenitor cell population contributing to osteoconduction, combining some autogenous bone into the graft composite is highly recommended. Three-, four-, and five-wall bony defects have a sufficient population of osteoprogenitor cells in close proximity so that they need only a small percentage of autogenous bone or none at all. In each situation, PRP has proven benefits, and in all such grafts, PRP's effect on the overlying flap will support capillary ingrowth and reduce dehiscence and bone extrusions.

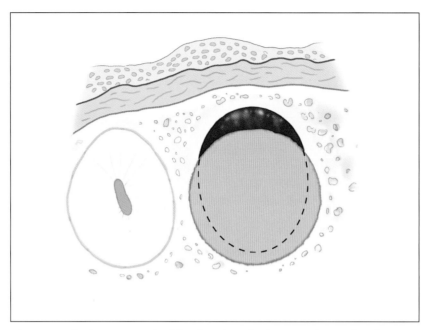

Fig 3-34a Placing an oversized implant in a fresh extraction socket does not eliminate the gap between the implant and the socket wall.

Alveolar Ridge Preservation

Preservation of bone and of bony contours after tooth removal allows for ideal implant positioning and optimal esthetics in both provisional and final restorations. Ridge preservation is important in all areas of the arches, but it is of critical importance in the so-called esthetic zone in the anterior maxilla. A variety of complications can make alveolar ridge preservation more difficult. For example, teeth fractured below the alveolar crest, brittle root canal–treated teeth, ankylosed roots, a thin buccal cortical plate, fenestrations, and fistulae involving the buccal plate all complicate removal of the remaining tooth structure while preserving the circumferential bone of the socket. Such challenges make the term *atraumatic tooth removal* an unrealistic concept in many cases. Nevertheless, teeth should be removed with a minimal amount of soft tissue reflection and bone removal. If possible, an intrasocket approach should be taken rather than a labial approach that requires reflection of a mucoperiosteal flap. Even a carefully reflected mucoperiosteal flap separates the periosteal blood supply from the bone and induces some scarring of the cambium layer of the periosteum. The result is a bone resorption-remodeling cycle related to this reflection that is less than a 100% replacement and eventuates in the loss of 0.5 to 1.5 mm of crestal bone.

If sufficient crown structure is available, the forceps should be seated as far apical as possible. For single-rooted teeth, use a rotational force to mobilize the tooth while supporting the buccal plate with digital pressure. For multi-rooted teeth, an elliptical-delivered force by the forceps is preferred over the more traditional buccolingual luxation. Even then, digital support of the buccal plate is recommended.

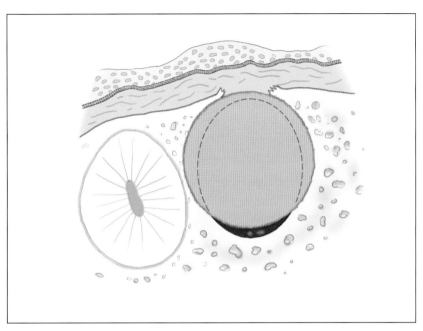

Fig 3-34b Placing an oversized implant along the central axis of the socket risks fenestrations through the buccal-cortical plate and risks damage to the adjacent root.

If there is insufficient crown structure to seat a forceps, or if the root is fractured below the alveolar crest, use a periotome or a no. 11 scalpel blade to sever the periodontal ligament fibers at the furthest apical extent possible. A thin-bladed elevator, such as a 301 or a root-tip elevator, can then be used as a wedge to displace and luxate the root. Should this approach prove unsuccessful, a deep slot can be placed in the root across its diameter with a 701 or 702 tapered fissure bur. Then the 301 elevator or a slotted screwdriver found in most bone plate and screw kits can be used to apply a rotation force for root removal, or the root itself can be sectioned and removed in pieces without compromising the bony circumference of the socket. Another approach is to seat an oversized root canal file (no. 80 or 100) in the pulp chamber and engage a sufficient amount of dentin. Use this as a handle on the root to supply a coronal vector of force, and use a root tip elevator to act as a wedge to remove the root without removing bone.

If the socket walls and native alveolar bone height can be maintained during tooth removal, no further procedures may be necessary. The soft tissue contours will be maintained and the socket can be expected to heal and spontaneously regenerate sufficient bone for implant placement within 4 to 6 months. If an immediate implant is used, do not attempt to fill the entire socket by using a large-diameter implant. Tooth sockets are oval, whereas dental implants are round; therefore, gaps of 0.1 to 3.0 mm will result between the implant and bone. Placing a wide-diameter implant will not eliminate these gaps and may outfracture the buccal plate (Fig 3-34a). Moreover, the central axis of the implant will be located too far to the buccal for an ideal restoration (Fig 3-34b). Place the

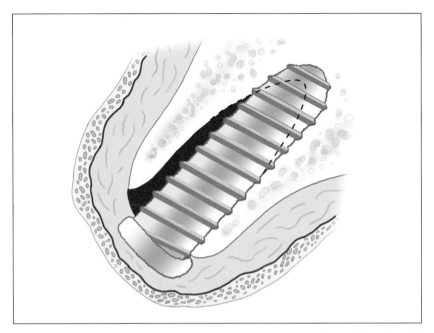

Fig 3-34c Immediate implants placed into fresh extraction sockets should engage the lingual/palatal cortex, be seated 3 mm apical to the socket apex, and emerge in the cingulum position.

standard-diameter implant recommended for the specific tooth position, that is, 3.25 mm for mandibular incisors and maxillary lateral incisors, 4.0 mm for canines and premolars, and 5.0 mm for molars and maxillary central incisors. For anterior teeth and premolars, however, the implant should not be placed through the apex of the socket in the long axis of the root. Instead, it should be placed slightly into the socket's lingual or palatal wall in order to engage more bone for primary stability (see Fig 3-34a). The implant should also be positioned so that its apex is located 3 mm apical and palatal/lingual to the apex of the socket (Fig 3-34c). By eliminating one gap area, the amount of direct bone-to-metal contact will also be increased and the implant emergence will be at the cingulum or lingual cusp position for an optimal restoration. Although the remaining implant-to–socket wall gaps may be slightly enlarged by this process, they will nonetheless be manageable.

For gaps of 2 mm or less, the authors recommend using PRP alone (Fig 3-35a). The growth factors in PRP will attach themselves to the cell membranes of the endosteal osteoblasts in the socket wall and to the marrow stem cells exposed to the socket, inducing proliferation of the former and differentiation of the latter into osteoblasts, and eventually producing bone in the gap (Figs 3-35b and 3-35c). Migration across the gap is facilitated by the fibrin-fibronectin-vitronectin cell adhesion molecules found in PRP; these adhesion molecules form a matrix along which the cells can simultaneously migrate, differentiate, and produce bone. This

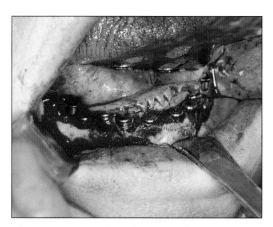

Fig 3-35a Immediate implant placement into extraction sockets does not require grafting if the gap between the implant and socket wall is 2 mm or less and PRP is used.

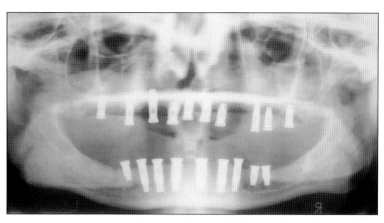

Fig 3-35b Bone regeneration into multiple extraction sockets with immediate implant placement.

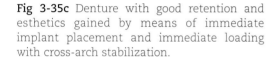

Fig 3-35c Denture with good retention and esthetics gained by means of immediate implant placement and immediate loading with cross-arch stabilization.

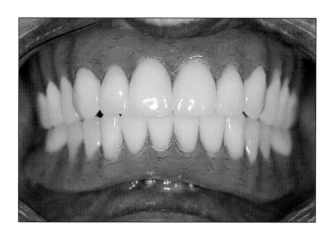

mechanism, which is detailed in chapter 1, describes the basic process of osteoconduction in all situations and applies even to gaps as great as 2 mm (see chapter 1, Figs 1-37a to 1-37d).

In cases where the gap is 2 mm or more, the authors recommend using a graft material of the clinician's choice together with PRP (Figs 3-36a and 3-36b). Since the socket wall is an adequate source of endosteal osteoblasts and marrow stem cells and the defect volume is relatively small, autogenous bone is not necessary. Allogeneic bone or bone substitutes, combined with PRP, will form an adequate matrix for osteoconduction through the same mechanisms described above for gaps that are less than 2 mm wide (Fig 3-36c). In the larger gaps, the graft material functions to maintain the fibrin-fibronectin-vitronectin matrix for a longer period of time to allow the osteoprogenitor cells to migrate a greater distance. In addition, the fibrin-fibronectin-vitronectin composite will adhere to the surfaces of the graft particles and the implant, forming a matrix on which bone can be deposited until the gap is filled and osseointegration is achieved.

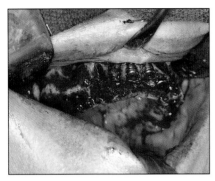

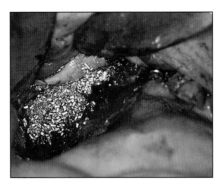

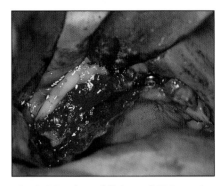

Fig 3-36a Immediate implant placement into extraction sockets with gaps between the implant and socket walls that measure greater than 2 mm or with loss of the buccal cortex requires grafting, PRP, and often a guided tissue regeneration membrane.

Fig 3-36b A composite of 30% autogenous cancellous marrow and 70% C-Graft is used to reconstruct the buccal cortical defects and the implant–socket wall gaps.

Fig 3-36c The addition of PRP to the composite graft shown in Fig 3-36b provides growth factors to the graft and facilitates adhesion of the graft particles into a form that can be contoured.

All too often, a so-called buccal wall blowout will cause the thin buccal plate to be lost (Fig 3-37a). Left untreated, it will result in a buccolingual deficiency that may make it impossible to place an implant and/or lead to an unesthetic concavity. When grafting of this defect is delayed, the only option available may be an autogenous onlay graft, which is more complex and is associated with a higher rate of morbidity than other grafting procedures. Therefore, immediate grafting is strongly recommended using allogeneic bone or bone substitutes to regenerate viable bone in the socket and maintain the buccal contour. In the esthetic zone, this situation takes on heightened importance, particularly if implants are planned.

The authors recommend combining activated PRP with particulate allogeneic nondemineralized bone (eg, Puros, PepGen P-15), a bone substitute (eg, C-Graft), or a xenogeneic graft (eg, Bio-Oss, Puros) and allowing the clot to mature for 1 minute. At the same time, a small amount of activated PRP should be placed into the socket and around the buccal plate. The easy-to-handle PRP-graft composite is then placed into the socket and molded to form an ideal buccal contour (Figs 3-37b and 3-37c). When using nonviable graft materials, tight packing is counterproductive and should be avoided. Nonviable grafts promote bone regeneration by mechanisms involving migration and ingrowth of bone from the surrounding walls and therefore require space between the particles for formation of an osteoconductive matrix. The cell adhesion molecules (fibrin, fibronectin, and vitronectin) in PRP supply this matrix, but packing of the graft particles too tightly may leave insufficient space for this osteoconductive matrix and result in fibrous ingrowth instead of bone. Therefore, the graft particles–PRP complex should loosely fill the defect and then be covered with a soft tissue primary closure (Figs 3-37d to 3-37f).

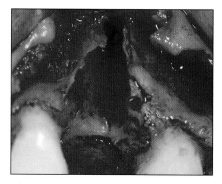

Fig 3-37a Loss of the buccal plate after an extraction results in a concavity and possible insufficient bone to place an implant. (Figs 3-37a to 3-37f courtesy of Dr Paul Petrungaro, Stillwater, Minnesota.)

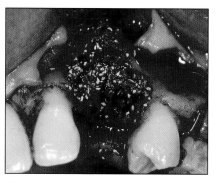

Fig 3-37b Socket preservation via grafting with a composite of PepGen P-15 and PRP.

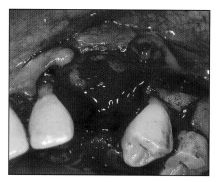

Fig 3-37c Additional PRP is placed as a membrane over the graft just prior to closure.

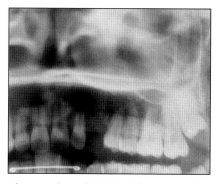

Fig 3-37d Radiograph of socket preservation graft.

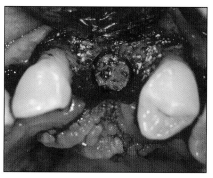

Fig 3-37e Core biopsy of graft during implant placement. Note the preservation of the canine eminence and the regeneration of bone in the socket.

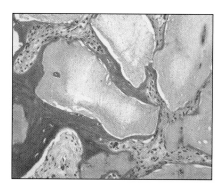

Fig 3-37f Histology of core biopsy from the socket preservation graft with PRP shows PepGen P-15 particles and bone in direct contact.

References

1. Marx RE, Carlson ER, Eichstaedt RM, Schimmele SR, Strauss JE, Georgeff K. Platelet-rich plasma—Growth factor enhancement for bone grafts. Oral Surg Oral Med Oral Pathol Oral Radiol Endod 1998;85:638–646.
2. Peleg M, Mazor Z, Garg AK. Augmentation grafting of the maxillary sinus and simultaneous implant placement in patients with 3 to 5 mm of residual alveolar bone height. Int J Oral Maxillofac Implants 1999;14:549–556.
3. Olson JW, Dent CD, Morris HF, Ochi S. Long-term assessment (5 to 71 months) of endosseous dental implants placed in the augmented maxillary sinus. Ann Periodontol 2000;5:152–156.
4. Mazor Z, Peleg M, Garg AK, Luboshitz J. Platelet-rich plasma for bone graft enhancement in sinus floor augmentation with simultaneous implant placement: Patient series study. Implant Dent 2004;13:65–72.

5. Schopper C, Moser D, Sabbas A, et al. The fluorohydroxyapatite (FHA) FRIOS Algipore is a suitable biomaterial for the reconstruction of severely atrophic human maxillae. Clin Oral Implants Res 2003;14:743–749.

6. Quinones CR, Hurzeler MB, Schupbach P, Arnold DR, Strub JR, Caffesse RG. Maxillary sinus augmentation using different grafting materials and dental implants in monkeys. Part IV. Evaluation of hydroxyapatite-coated implants. Clin Oral Implants Res 1997;8:497–505.

7. Landi L, Pretel RW Jr, Hakimi NM, Setayesh R. Maxillary sinus floor elevation using a combination of DFDBA and bovine-derived porous hydroxyapatite: A preliminary histologic and histomorphometric report. Int J Periodontics Restorative Dent 2000;20:574–583.

8. Haas R, Baron M, Donath K, Zechner W, Watzek G. Porous hydroxyapatite for grafting the maxillary sinus: A comparative histomorphometric study in sheep. Int J Oral Maxillofac Implants 2002;17:337–346.

9. Shlomi B, Horowitz I, Kahn A, Dobriyan A, Chaushu G. The effect of sinus membrane perforation and repair with Lambone on the outcome of maxillary sinus floor augmentation: A radiographic assessment. Int J Oral Maxillofac Implants 2004;19:559–562.

10. Marx RE. Platelet-rich plasma: A source of multiple autogenous growth factors for bone grafts. In: Lynch SE, Genco RJ, Marx RE (eds). Tissue Engineering: Applications in Maxillofacial Surgery and Periodontics. Chicago: Quintessence, 1999:71–82.

11. Field EA, Speechley JA, Rotter E, Scott J. Dry socket incidence compared after a 12 year interval. Br J Oral Maxillofac Surg 1985;23:419–427.

12. Heasman PA, Jacobs DJ. A clinical investigation into the incidence of dry socket. Br J Oral Maxillofac Surg 1984;22:115–122.

13. Babbush CA. The use of PRP in conjunction with other bone graft materials: Allograft, alloplast, xenograft. Presented at the 2nd Symposium on Platelet-Rich Plasma (PRP) & Its Growth Factors, San Francisco, 23–26 Apr 2003.

14. Mancuso J, Bennion JW, Hull MJ, Winterholler BW. Platelet-rich plasma: A preliminary report in routine impacted mandibular third molar surgery and the prevention of alveolar osteitis. J Oral Maxillofacial Surg 2003;61(suppl 1).

15. Nyman S. Bone regeneration using the principle of guided tissue regeneration. J Clin Periodontol 1991;18:494–498.

16. Lekovic V, Camargo PM, Weinlaender M, Vasilic N, Aleksic Z, Kenney EB. Effectiveness of a combination of platelet-rich plasma, bovine porous bone mineral and guided tissue regeneration in the treatment of mandibular grade II molar furcations in humans. J Clin Periodontol 2003;30:746–751.

17. Camargo PM, Lekovic V, Weinlaender M, Vasilic N, Madzarevic M, Kenney EB. Platelet-rich plasma and bovine porous bone mineral combined with guided tissue regeneration in the treatment of intrabony defects in humans. J Periodontal Res 2002;37:300–306.

18. Lekovic V, Camargo PM, Weinlaender M, Vasilic N, Kenney EB. Comparison of platelet-rich plasma, bovine porous bone mineral, and guided tissue regeneration versus platelet-rich plasma and bovine porous bone mineral in the treatment of intrabony defects: A reentry study. J Periodontol 2002;73:198–205.

19. Kim SG, Chung CH, Kim YK, Park JC, Lim SC. Use of particulate dentin-plaster of Paris combination with/without platelet-rich plasma in the treatment of bone defects around implants. Int J Oral Maxillofac Implants 2002;17:86–94.

20. Kovacs K, Velich N, Huszar T, et al. Comparative study of beta-tricalcium phosphate mixed with platelet-rich plasma versus beta-tricalcium phosphate, a bone substitute material in dentistry. Acta Vet Hung 2003;51:475–484.

21. Kassolis JD, Rosen PS, Reynolds MA. Alveolar ridge and sinus augmentation utilizing platelet-rich plasma in combination with freeze-dried bone allograft: Case series. J Periodontol 2000;71:1654–1661.

22. Marx RE, Snyder R, Kline SN. Cellular survival of human marrow during placement of marrow-cancellous bone grafts. J Oral Surg 1979;37:712–718.

chapter four

Regeneration of Soft Tissue in Dental Procedures

Since the early 1990s, the need to enhance soft tissue healing has taken on much greater importance. Today, wound care centers treat chronic nonhealing wounds using growth factor technology and the concept of an improved wound environment. Cosmetic surgeons are treating ever-increasing numbers of patients requesting facial soft tissue surgery. Oral and maxillofacial surgeons and periodontists have developed predictable techniques for using free gingival and connective tissue grafts for indications such as root-coverage procedures and esthetic refinements in implant therapy, while general dental practitioners routinely use several types of soft tissue flaps and grafts for a variety of indications.

The use of platelet-rich plasma (PRP) to enhance soft tissue healing has earned an established role in a wide variety of soft tissue procedures across several disciplines. In facial cosmetic surgery, it is being used to reduce swelling and ecchymosis and to speed healing in traditional face lifts, blepharoplasties, and laser skin resurfacing.[1] In dermatologic surgery, it is being used to gain faster and more complete healing with less scarring after excision of skin lesions.[2] In cardiac surgery, it has reduced the incidence of sternal wound dehiscences and delayed healing.[3] In wound care centers, it has achieved healing of refractory diabetic ulcers and ulcers due to peripheral vascular disease[4] (Figs 4-1a to 4-1f). Each of these disciplines has witnessed improved outcomes with PRP use (Figs 4-2a to 4-2c). This chapter focuses on specific soft tissue procedures in periodontal and implant surgery that are enhanced by the use of PRP.

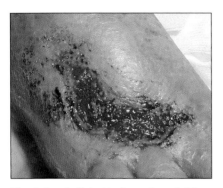

Fig 4-1a A diabetic foot ulcer, initiated by neuropathy, progresses because of microangiopathy and can lead to amputation. (Figs 4-1a to 4-1e courtesy of Dr Jürgen Becker, Düsseldorf, Germany.)

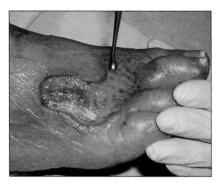

Fig 4-1b Careful debridement of the wound is the first step.

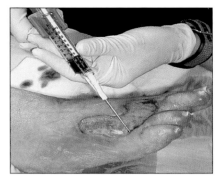

Fig 4-1c PRP is used topically to facilitate healing, thus helping to prevent an amputation.

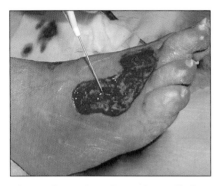

Fig 4-1d Activated PRP is applied to the surface of the wound prior to covering it with an Opsite dressing (Smith & Nephew).

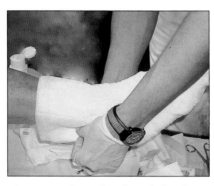

Fig 4-1e A loose bandage helps keep the PRP in place and prevent additional contamination.

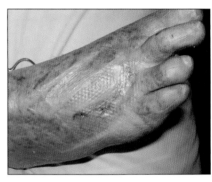

Fig 4-1f Taken 4 months after treatment with PRP, this photo shows the rapid and nearly complete healing that was apparent as early as 4 weeks. (Courtesy of Dr G. Friese, Düsseldorf, Germany.)

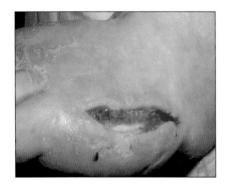

Fig 4-2a Another diabetic ulcer illustrates how bony prominences of the foot are the most vulnerable areas in these patients. PRP was used to facilitate healing after initial wound care of this ulcer. (Figs 4-2a and 4-2b courtesy of Dr Jürgen Becker, Düsseldorf, Germany.)

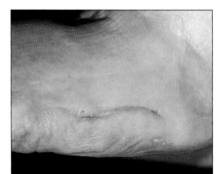

Fig 4-2b The ulcer shows the positive effects of initial wound care and application of PRP. The ulcer is nearly healed, and the pain and swelling have resolved.

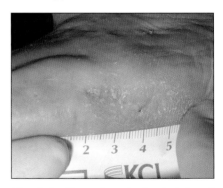

Fig 4-2c The ulcer is healed by 6 weeks. (Courtesy of Dr G. Friese, Düsseldorf, Germany.)

Soft Tissue Flaps During Implant Surgery

In placing dental implants, surgeons usually take for granted that the flap will heal, its blood supply will be intact, and the periosteum has good osteogenic potential. The reality, however, is that patients who require dental implants are likely to have lost soft tissue and the osteogenic capability of the periosteum, as well as teeth. The long-term inflammation associated with chronic periodontitis leads to scarring of the periosteum and therefore loss of its osteogenic potential. The periosteum is further scarred and the blood supply altered by the physical removal of the tooth, particularly when a mucoperiosteal flap is reflected. The periosteum and the full thickness of the mucosa may also have been compromised by dental abscesses, apicoectomies, repeated periodontal surgeries, and especially by grafting procedures using nonviable graft materials, all of which reduce the soft tissue blood supply and the osteogenic capability of the periosteum. Healing can be even further compromised by external factors and agents such as smoking or the use of smokeless tobacco, steroid medication, or radiation therapy, and by systemic diseases such as diabetes, peripheral vascular disease, or systemic lupus erythematosis. In addition, advanced age is also known to reduce the rate and degree of healing. For all of these reasons, PRP has a strong potential in implant flap surgery, regardless of the particular type of flap employed.

The full-thickness mucoperiosteal flap elevated from a crestal incision is the standard flap used to place dental implants. Alternative flap designs, such as those elevated from a buccally or palatally placed incision, or the vascularized periosteal–connective tissue flap, have also been used. Since the periosteum is likely to be compromised by previous disease and/or surgeries regardless of flap design, PRP is recommended for all such flaps. Upon reflection, the flap will contract and therefore resist advancement for a tension-free closure. Since the periosteum does not contribute significantly to bone regeneration in these situations, the surgeon should not hesitate to incise the periosteum and undermine the mucosa in a plane superficial to any muscle attachments (Fig 4-3a). By this means, the flap can be closed primarily with eversion to maximize healing (Fig 4-3b). In addition, undermining the flap to separate it from any facial muscle attachments will prevent microseparations in the closure and hence leakage of saliva during lip and cheek movements.

Activated PRP is applied either to the undersurface of the flap or over the bone and implant just prior to closure (Figs 4-4a to 4-4c). This will accomplish a seal at the suture line, which will also resist leakage. PRP's mechanism of action in this application is that the growth factors will speed the rate of vascular ingrowth into the bone, thereby reducing the degree and risk of crestal bone loss, and the cell adhesion molecules will initially stabilize the flap and help seal the closure, then later serve as a matrix for osteoconduction and vascular ingrowth (Figs 4-4d and 4-4e).

Although PRP is an option in stage 2 implant-uncovering procedures, it is not essential unless numerous implants are to be uncovered and the mucosa has been severely compromised by repeated surgeries, infections, previously failed grafting procedures, or radiation therapy.

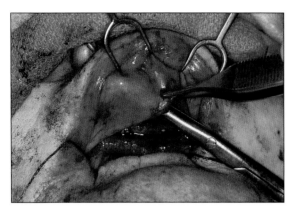

Fig 4-3a The mucosa must be extensively undermined in a superficial plane, separating muscle attachments from the mucosa.

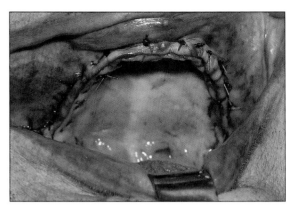

Fig 4-3b Flap closure should include eversion of the edges, accomplished here with a horizontal mattress suture.

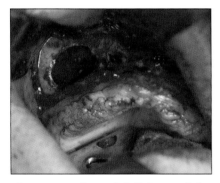

Fig 4-4a Horizontal deficiency of the maxilla and sinus lift surgical site prepared for grafting.

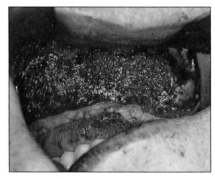

Fig 4-4b Composite graft made of autogenous bone and a bone substitute (C-Graft, The Clinician's Preference) placed into sinus lift site and onlaid onto the horizontal maxillary deficiency.

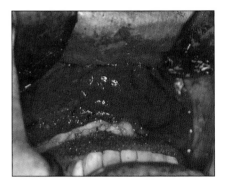

Fig 4-4c Activated PRP is applied over the composite graft and on the undersurface of the flap.

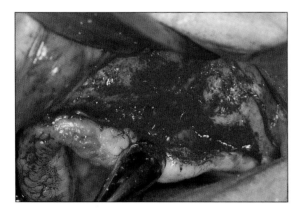

Fig 4-4d Upon re-entry at 4 months, the graft has matured and consolidated.

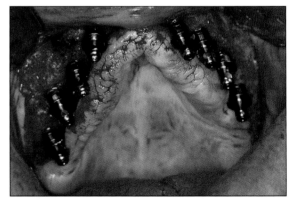

Fig 4-4e Mature graft with sufficient density for primary stability of implants.

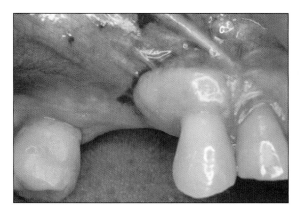

Fig 4-5a Missing attached gingiva in an edentulous area can be replaced with an autologous soft tissue graft of keratinized mucosa.

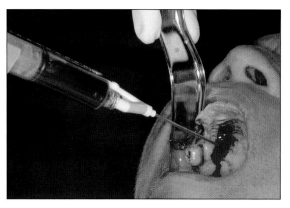

Fig 4-5b Keratinized mucosa is usually obtained from the palate. PRP is applied to combat the bleeding that can result from this tissue harvest as well as to enhance its healing.

Fig 4-5c Coating the donor area with PRP helps achieve hemostasis and enhances healing time and comfort.

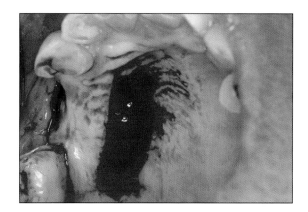

Free Gingival Grafts

Free gingival grafts are used to cover a root dehiscence or an implant exposure, to release a high mucogingival attachment, or to improve tissue appearance in the esthetic zone. The outcome of these procedures is readily apparent to the patient and to any referring dentist and will be held up to scrutiny by both. Therefore, this apparently simple and minor procedure carries a strong indication for healing enhancement.

The most common application for a free gingival graft is to increase the zone of attached tissue caused by recession or a high mucogingival attachment (Fig 4-5a). For this procedure, keratinized mucosa is harvested from the palate in the area of the lateral palatal shelf adjacent to the molar and premolar teeth. Because of the rich vascularity and nerve density in this area, excessive postoperative bleeding and significant pain may be experienced by the patient. To combat this, electrocautery is recommended for coagulation, and the use of activated platelet-poor plasma (PPP) or even PRP is recommended for hemostasis (Figs 4-5b and 4-5c). Some practitioners even suture a small compression bolster over the area, but this is generally not required.

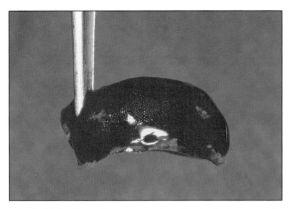

Fig 4-5d Before placement, the gingival tissue graft is internally coated with PRP.

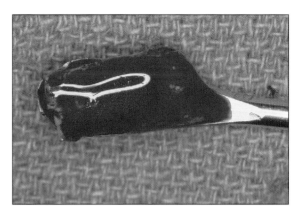

Fig 4-5e Since PRP growth factors are released quickly, the graft should be coated just prior to placement.

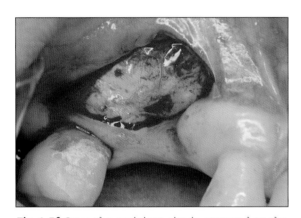

Fig 4-5f Once the recipient site is prepared to the periosteal level, a coating of PRP can be applied.

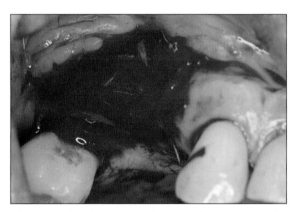

Fig 4-5g After the free gingival graft is placed, another coating of PRP is applied.

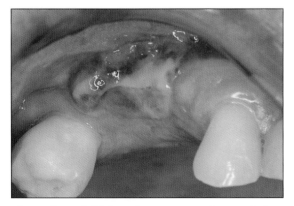

Fig 4-5h An initial graft acceptance is revealed at suture removal 7 days later. Note correction of the mucogingival banding.

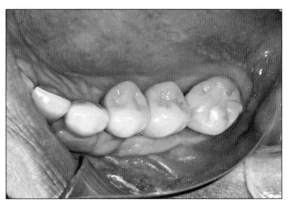

Fig 4-5i The matured gingival graft developed a normal vestibule and gained a normal-appearing attached gingiva.

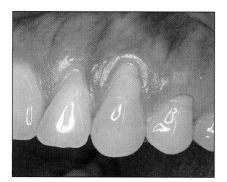

Fig 4-6a Abrasive brushing habits can cause recession of the vulnerable thin mucosa over the canine prominence.

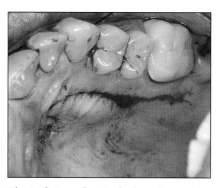

Fig 4-6b A pocket technique is used to remove connective tissue from under the surface epithelium, between the alveolar and palatal processes, leaving it intact for suturing and avoiding a denuded wound.

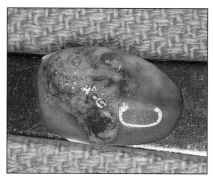

Fig 4-6c The palatal connective tissue is covered with PRP just before placement at the recipient site.

The authors recommend placing the harvested full-thickness gingival graft in activated PRP (Figs 4-5d and 4-5e) while the recipient site is being prepared. This will allow the growth factors in PRP to be secreted and to attach themselves to the membranes of the cells in the graft, while the cell adhesion molecules coat the deep surface of the graft. Both of these mechanisms will facilitate adhesion of the graft to the recipient site and then promote the capillary and connective tissue ingrowth necessary for complete survival of the graft (Figs 4-5f to 4-5i).

Connective Tissue Grafts

A growing interest in esthetic dentistry over the past decade has made connective tissue grafting a relatively common procedure. Today it is often used to create or add bulk and contour to the labial gingiva around a natural tooth or an implant-retained crown. It may also be used for root coverage in cases of slight or moderate root exposure (Fig 4-6a). It is frequently used in the esthetic zone to create a more natural-appearing gingiva-tooth interface.

The connective tissue used in this procedure is almost always harvested from the lateral palatal shelf opposite the molars and premolars. In contrast to free gingival grafts harvested from the same area, the connective tissue graft donor site is closed primarily and therefore has less postoperative bleeding and pain (Fig 4-6b). Placing PRP in this donor site is thus optional since the rich vascularity of the tissue and the use of a primary closure usually result in rapid and uncomplicated healing. However, like the free gingival graft, the connective tissue graft should be incubated in activated PRP while the recipient site is prepared (Fig 4-6c). This will allow the platelets to secrete their seven growth factors that will attach to the membranes of the cells in the graft as the graft's collagen fibrils become coated with the cell adhesion molecules in PRP.

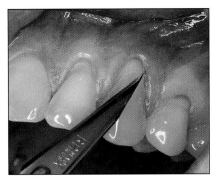

Fig 4-6d In a tunneling fashion, periodontal fibers are carefully dissected 1 to 3 mm apically, leaving the most incisal attachments of the papillae intact.

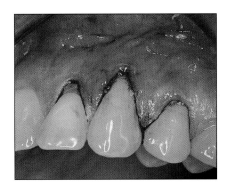

Fig 4-6e In this tunneling procedure, both the mesial and distal papillae of the canine are tunneled through but left attached at the crest.

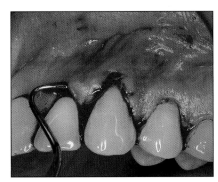

Fig 4-6f Periodontal probes and similar instruments are useful for both detaching the fibers and assessing the adequacy of the dissection.

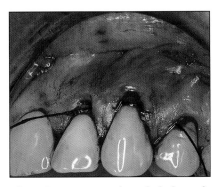

Fig 4-6g A suture, threaded through the tunneled gingival tissue, is pulled up and down to help assess the correct undermining of the area.

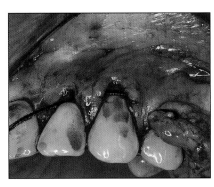

Fig 4-6h The suture is then placed through the connective tissue at an adequate distance from its edge to avoid tearing as it is pulled through the tunnel.

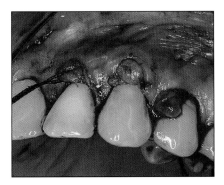

Fig 4-6i The graft tissue is carefully pulled through the gingival tunnel and placed in the desired position. PRP helps the graft incorporate (attach) earlier, correcting the tissue recession.

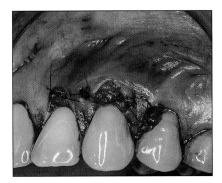

Fig 4-6j A small-diameter (5.0 or 6.0) nylon suture is recommended to hold this minuscule graft in place. All phases of this procedure should be done with utmost care since the recipient site and the graft are relatively small.

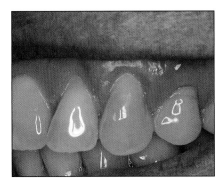

Fig 4-6k After 1 month, the gingival recession is resolved. PRP's enhancement of graft incorporation and healing contributed greatly to this root coverage.

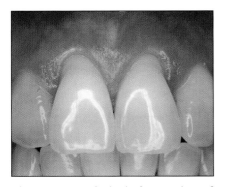

Fig 4-7a Buccal gingival recession of the two maxillary central incisors exposes almost one fourth of the root, compromising esthetics and promoting sensitivity to heat and cold. (Figs 4-7a to 4-7h courtesy of Dr Paul Petrungaro, Minneapolis, MN.)

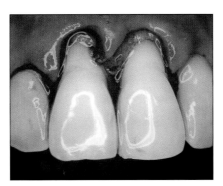

Fig 4-7b A sulcular incision on the buccal surface of both central incisors is followed by slight flap elevation to expose the roots an additional 2 to 3 mm.

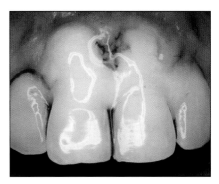

Fig 4-7c An EDTA solution is applied to the exposed root surface to remove proteinaceous debris and to open the dentinal tubules.

The root surface should be prepared using a saturated solution of citric acid, a solution of tetracycline hydrochloride, or ethylenediaminetetraacetic acid (EDTA). This removes any proteinaceous deposits from the root surface and etches the dentin, opening the dentinal tubules for maximum ingrowth of the graft and development of a firm fibrous attachment to the root. Once the root surface has been debrided and etched in this fashion, the authors recommend coating it with activated PRP.

The soft tissue component of the recipient site is usually developed by means of an interproximal papilla–sparing sulcular incision and dissection (Figs 4-6d to 4-6f). The purpose of this tunneling procedure is to elevate the mucosa from the periosteum and gain a volume space to accommodate the graft. The PRP-coated connective tissue graft is then pulled through the tunnel from one end to the other using a 3-0 silk suture (Figs 4-6g to 4-6i). The mucosa is then coronally repositioned and sutured to the palatal mucosa to achieve maximum stabilization (Fig 4-6j). This procedure will serve to increase the gingival contour for improved esthetics as well as to cover the exposed root (Fig 4-6k). Overcontouring of the graft is unnecessary since the rapid revascularization promoted by PRP will maintain the viability of the transplanted cells and prevent shrinkage. As with the other soft tissue procedures discussed in this chapter, stabilizing the graft is critical for complete integration and a precise outcome. Trauma to the graft or even micromotion will shear off the new capillaries growing into the graft and disrupt collagen formation that would otherwise ensure its incorporation. Despite its capacity to accelerate these phases of the healing process, PRP cannot compensate for the effects of trauma or disruption of the graft. Like any adjunct to healing, PRP will supplement but will not replace good basic surgical principles, which together will speed healing, reduce pain, and produce a better quality of tissue (Figs 4-7a to 4-7h).

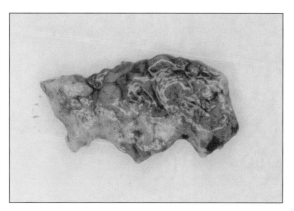

Fig 4-7d The connective tissue graft should be shaped to conform to the natural gingival contours and embrasures.

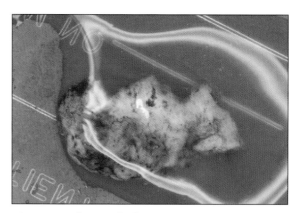

Fig 4-7e Before graft placement, both the graft and the recipient site are thoroughly coated with PRP.

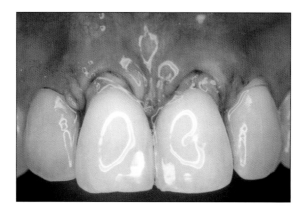

Fig 4-7f The grafted tissue is sutured securely to prevent micromovements that could disrupt vascularity and collagen formation enhanced by PRP. The gingival flap is then advanced coronally to cover the graft.

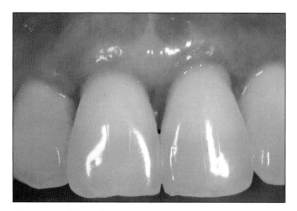

Fig 4-7g The soft tissues healed after only 3 weeks, providing optimal root coverage.

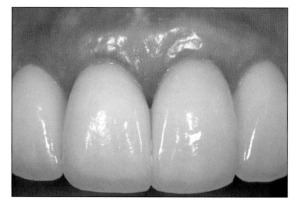

Fig 4-7h Effective soft tissue healing motivated the patient to seek further improvement in esthetics through veneer fabrication.

Coronally Repositioned Flaps and Allogeneic Dermis for Root Coverage

A technique recently developed for root coverage in cases where an excessive amount of root exposure has occurred has produced dramatic results (Figs 4-8a and 4-8b). This technique combines the use of two materials—allogeneic human dermis (AlloDerm, LifeCell) and PRP—with a coronally repositioned flap to achieve a predictable outcome.

In this approach, the allogeneic dermis is rehydrated in activated PRP (rather than the standard saline) while the root surface is prepared with a saturated citric acid solution or other agent and the full-thickness flap is reflected (Fig 4-8c). The allogeneic dermis is then placed over the root surfaces (usually several adjacent roots are involved and treated simultaneously) and the bone (Fig 4-8d). It is then trimmed to follow the curvature of the gingival margin and sutured through the interproximal spaces to the lingual or palatal gingiva (Figs 4-8e and 4-8f). The apical edge is often tacked to bone using the tacks designed to secure a barrier membrane. Activated PRP is applied to the affixed allogeneic dermis and to the undersurface of the mucoperiosteal flap before it is sutured (Fig 4-8g).

This approach has been successful in covering multiple roots where each has a significant degree of exposure. Other approaches, such as free gingival grafts and local flaps, are less efficacious for this indication because of the limited availability of donor tissue and/or morbidity and scarring at the donor site. The results of a split-mouth study using an allogeneic dermis rehydrated with saline on one side and an allogeneic dermis rehydrated and covered with PRP on the other revealed less swelling, less inflammation, and less pain, with no exposure of the allogeneic dermis on the PRP-treated side as compared with the opposite side.[5,6] The purpose of the allogeneic dermis is to promote healing of the coronally repositioned flap in its new location without undergoing apical retraction. To do so, it must first adhere to and become integrated with the bone adjacent to the exposed roots, thus functioning as periosteum. The coronally repositioned flap must then heal and adhere to this substitute "periosteum" before wound-healing contraction occurs. The need for the allogeneic dermis to adhere to and be rapidly incorporated into the bone adjacent to these exposed roots is therefore critical to the outcome of this procedure. PRP's cell adhesion molecules—fibrin, fibronectin, and vitronectin—assist in the initial adherence and act as a scaffold for the rapid incorporation of the allogeneic dermis to bone as well as to the coronally repositioned flap. As with each of the other soft tissue procedures, the seven growth factors in PRP will also promote capillary and connective tissue ingrowth into the allogeneic dermis from the underlying bone as well as from the overlying coronally repositioned flap. Therefore, the composite of allogeneic dermis, PRP, and a full-thickness mucoperiosteal flap heals to the repositioned location and achieves coverage even in the most advanced cases of root exposure (Figs 4-9a to 4-9e).

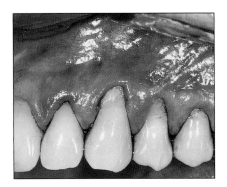

Fig 4-8a Gingival recession results in root exposure that is most severe in the areas around the maxillary canine and adjacent premolars. (Figs 4-8a to 4-8g courtesy of Dr Edward P. Allen, Dallas, Texas.)

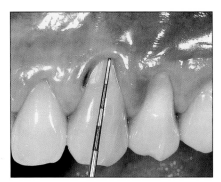

Fig 4-8b A periodontal probe measures 3 mm of undesirable root exposure in the canine area.

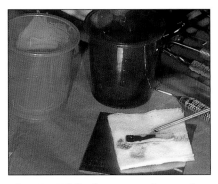

Fig 4-8c While the root surface undergoes preparation with citric acid, the allogeneic dermal tissue is rehydrated with PRP instead of the standard saline solution.

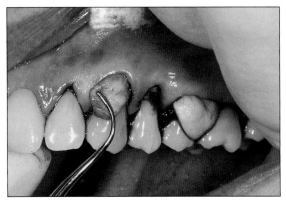

Fig 4-8d A full-thickness flap facilitates placement of the allogeneic dermis onto the bone and root surfaces.

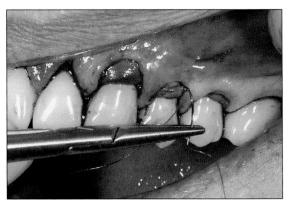

Fig 4-8e The dermal tissue is sutured securely in place to ensure immobility during the healing process.

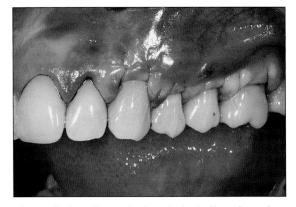

Fig 4-8f The allogeneic dermis is scallop-shaped to the correct height using special periodontal scalpel blades immediately before it is sutured into place.

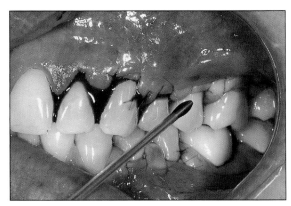

Fig 4-8g The complete surgical area is covered with PRP so that its growth factors can be released after suturing.

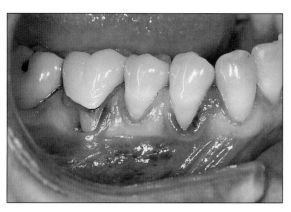

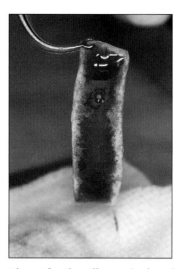

Fig 4-9a The roots are exposed in the right mandibular quadrant, including the canine, the two premolars, and, more severely, the mesial root of the first molar. (Figs 4-9a to 4-9e courtesy of Dr Edward P. Allen, Dallas, Texas.)

Fig 4-9b The allogeneic dermis is shaped to completely fill in the soft tissue defect. A comparable amount of soft tissue graft harvested from the oral cavity would cause significant morbidity.

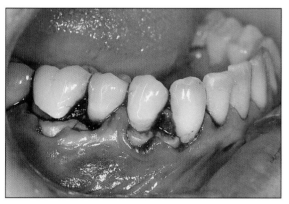

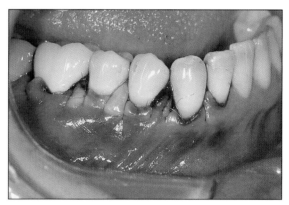

Fig 4-9c The soft tissue graft is evenly distributed under the reflected flap to cover the roots.

Fig 4-9d The surgical area is covered with PRP immediately before it is sutured to ensure immobility of the graft and overlying flap.

Fig 4-9e PRP used with an allogeneic human dermis graft can produce excellent results in as little as 3 weeks.

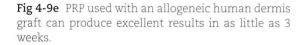

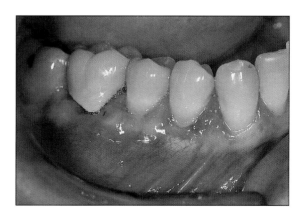

References

1. Powell DM, Chang E, Farrior EH. Recovery from deep-plane rhytidectomy following unilateral wound treatment with autologous platelet gel: A pilot study. Arch Facial Plast Surg 2001;3:245–250.
2. Adler SC, Kent KJ. Enhancing wound healing with growth factors. Facial Plast Surg Clin North Am 2002;10:129–146.
3. Stover EP, Siegel LC, Hood PA, O'Riordan GE, McKenna TR. Platelet-rich plasma sequestration, with therapeutic platelet yields, reduces allogeneic transfusion in complex cardiac surgery. Anesth Analg 2000;90:509–516.
4. Bennett SP, Griffiths GD, Schor AM, Leese GP, Schor SL. Growth factors in the treatment of diabetic foot ulcers. Br J Surg 2003;90:133–146.
5. Vastardis S, Yukna RA, Mayer ET. Platelet rich plasma plus AlloDerm for gingival recession treatment [abstract #1151]. J Dent Res 2004;83(special issue A).
6. Yukna RA. The performance of PRP with AlloDerm and gingival and mucosal flaps. Presented at the 2nd Symposium on Platelet-Rich Plasma (PRP) & Its Growth Factors, San Francisco, 23–26 Apr 2003.

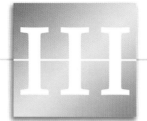
CRANIOFACIAL APPLICATIONS OF PLATELET-RICH PLASMA

Reconstruction of Major Tumor- and Trauma-Related Defects

Platelet-rich plasma (PRP) was first reported to enhance bone regeneration in major jaw reconstruction. Its initial scientific publication documented an accelerated rate of bone formation and increased bone density in continuity defects of the human jaw.[1] Since then, PRP's efficacy has also been documented in sinus lift grafts of all types,[2,3] bony ridge augmentations,[2,3] periodontal defect grafting,[4] third molar socket bone regeneration,[5] and several soft tissue healing applications.[6,7] Yet, large-scale bone grafting for mandibular and maxillary reconstruction remains one of its most important indications.

Mandibular Reconstruction

Extensive documentation of PRP's enhancement of autogenous cancellous marrow grafts is provided in chapter 1. The basic concept of autogenous marrow grafting is transplantation of endosteal osteoblasts and marrow stem cells, which are the osteoprogenitor cells that will regenerate bone in the defect. As noted in the chapters on sinus lift and ridge augmentation grafting, the surgeon should seek to increase the density of osteoprogenitor cells, first via mechanical syringe compaction and second via hand instrument compaction. PRP's role is to increase the number of osteoprogenitor cells via the mitogenic effects of the three platelet-derived growth factor (PDGF) isomers; to guide their differentiation toward and stimulate bone formation via the transforming growth factor beta (TGFβ) isomers; to stimulate early revascularization of the graft and hence greater

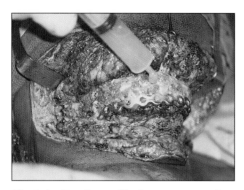

Fig 5-1a Total mandibular reconstruction with autogenous cancellous marrow contained by a rigid reconstruction plate. The surface is coated with PRP.

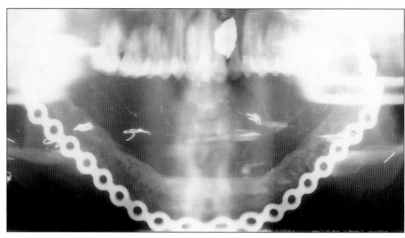

Fig 5-1b Radiographically consolidated bone graft enhanced by PRP at 3 months.

cellular survival and proliferation via the vascular endothelial growth factor (VEGF); and to promote osteoconduction from the host bone and throughout the graft via the cell adhesion molecules of fibrin, fibronectin, and vitronectin.

Today, cancellous marrow grafts for mandibular reconstruction are placed in one of three types of crib containments: allogeneic bone cribs, rigid titanium reconstruction plates, and, less commonly, titanium basket cribs. For each type of containment, the process of mechanical compaction of the cancellous marrow followed by hand instrument compaction is the same.

The application of PRP requires 60 mL of autologous blood to produce 7 to 10 mL of PRP with a platelet count of at least 1 million platelets/µL. Some surgeons recommend incubating the cancellous marrow in PRP prior to placement; the present authors do not since the cancellous marrow will be mechanically compacted within a syringe that can express some of the graft's growth factors and most of its cell adhesion molecules. Instead, the authors recommend placing the graft one section at a time, adding a small volume of activated PRP to each section. A small amount of PRP should be reserved to place over the surface of the graft once it is placed (Figs 5-1a and 5-1b). In this grafting approach and PRP application, the uppermost layer of activated PRP is of critical importance because the PRP-related growth factors from this layer seep into the graft as they are secreted by the platelets. Moreover, the cell adhesion molecules from this layer also trickle through the graft to interconnect the trabecular bone with strands of fibrin, fibronectin, and vitronectin to promote osteoconduction. When used in this manner, PRP accelerates the rate of bone regeneration and produces a sufficient bone density so that, as early as 3 months later, pre-prosthetic second surgeries, including dental implant placements (Fig 5-1c), split-thickness skin graft vestibuloplasties (Fig 5-1d), free gingival grafts, and alveoloplasties may be accomplished. The reader may recall from chapter 1 that PRP accelerates the rate of bone regeneration and improves bone density by 20%. However, it should be noted that PRP will not negate the effects of instability on a graft or the effects

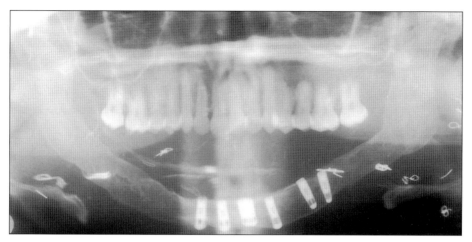

Fig 5-1c Dental implants placed into bone graft as early as 3 months.

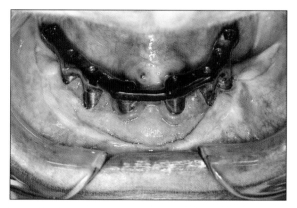

Fig 5-1d Split-thickness skin graft vestibuloplasty creates a vestibule and ridge to support a denture.

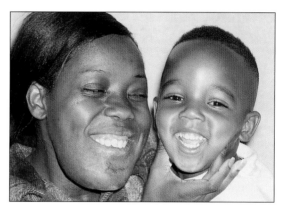

Fig 5-1e Complete mandibular reconstruction in this mother contributed to a normal appearance and family-oriented lifestyle.

of contamination. Each will render the graft nonviable. Instability prevents capillary ingrowth so that the graft fails to revascularize, the osteoprogenitor cells die, and the graft resorbs. Microorganisms directly lyse the osteoprogenitor cells, which also leads to graft resorption. Therefore, a contamination-free surgery and absolute graft stability for 4 to 6 weeks are the basic principles for predictable major jaw reconstruction that PRP can further enhance (Fig 5-1e).

Maxillary and Midface Reconstruction

Maxillary reconstruction

Maxillary reconstruction for tumor- and trauma-related defects generally does not require the use of a crib containment system. Although the maxillary denture-bearing surface may sometimes require a titanium basket crib, an autogenous

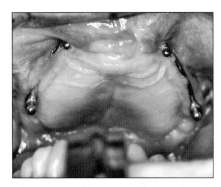

Fig 5-2a Failing maxillary subperiosteal implant with chronic long-term infection.

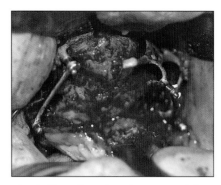

Fig 5-2b Infected subperiosteal implants such as these must be removed to resolve the infection.

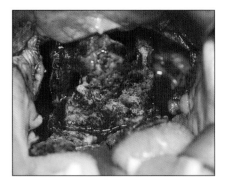

Fig 5-2c Nearly all the maxilla is lost due to the subperiosteal implant and its related trauma and infection.

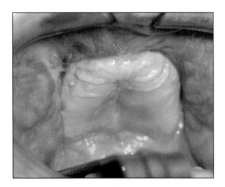

Fig 5-2d The maxilla can be reconstructed once the infection resolves. However, the soft tissue loss becomes evident as the wound contracts.

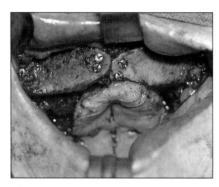

Fig 5-2e Autogenous corticocancellous block grafts lag-screwed to the host maxilla with a layer of PRP placed in between.

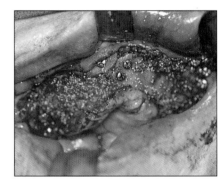

Fig 5-2f Additional autogenous cancellous marrow is placed between and around the block grafts.

block corticocancellous graft lag-screwed to the host bone and supplemented with additional cancellous marrow is more commonly used (Figs 5-2a to 5-2f). Because the maxilla is nonmobile, these grafts do not require maxillomandibular fixation. However, the graft must be rigidly fixated to the host maxilla and protected from denture trauma and/or occlusal forces for 4 to 6 weeks. The authors recommend placing a small amount of activated PRP on the surface of the maxilla just prior to lag-screw fixation of the graft. This will serve to incorporate the graft into the maxilla more rapidly.

Once the graft is placed, PRP should be applied to its surface (Fig 5-2g). Although incubating the graft in PRP can be beneficial, the surgeon should take care to reserve sufficient PRP for a final covering of the graft surface prior to closing, as in the protocol for mandibular reconstruction. Maxillary reconstruction differs from mandibular reconstruction in one fundamental respect. Maxillary bone graft reconstruction is accomplished via a transoral approach as compared to the extraoral transcutaneous approach required in most mandibular continuity reconstructions. A transoral approach is possible because *(1)* the maxilla is not a mobile bone, *(2)* its blood supply is greater, and *(3)* the graft volume/dead space is smaller. Each of these factors promotes a rapid revascularization and a resistance to infection, thereby allowing the graft to regenerate bone despite its placement into

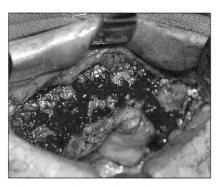

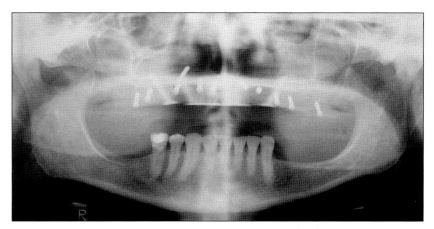

Fig 5-2g A layer of PRP is applied to the entire surface of the graft.

Fig 5-2h Panoramic radiograph showing the bone height gained by the graft and the graft's fixation with multiple lag screws.

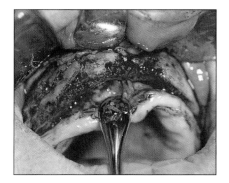

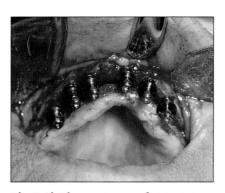

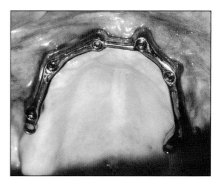

Fig 5-2i Upon re-entry and removal of the screws, the bone graft is found to be completely incorporated into the native maxilla and to have good arch form.

Fig 5-2j The mature graft accommodates ideal dental implant placement.

Fig 5-2k A Hader bar is used to connect the implants and act as a retentive mechanism for a maxillary appliance.

Fig 5-2l Because of the maturity of the bone graft and the well-integrated dental implants, a palateless denture can be fabricated.

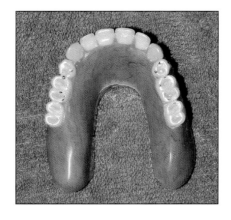

a contaminated tissue. The critical factors in maxillary reconstruction include stabilizing the graft, which may be accomplished using lag screws, a 1.5-mm plate, or a 2.0-mm plate (Fig 5-2h); thoroughly undermining the mucosa for an absolutely tension-free closure; and restricting denture wearing for a minimum of 4 to 6 weeks (Figs 5-2i to 5-2l).

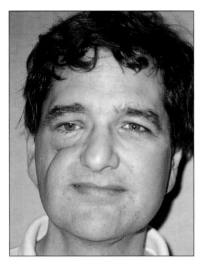

Fig 5-3a Facial indentation and cosmetic deformity related to a hemi-maxillectomy.

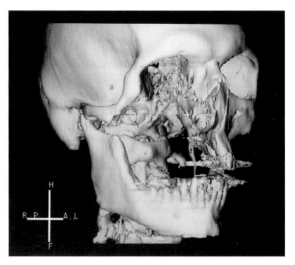

Fig 5-3b A significant amount of bone is missing from the maxilla, zygoma, and orbital floor.

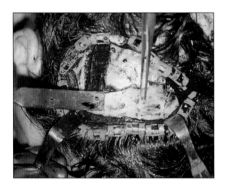

Fig 5-3c Split calvarial bone grafts are harvested from the parietal bone.

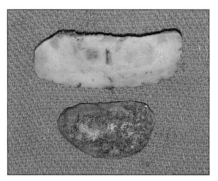

Fig 5-3d Calvarial bone grafts have a convex-concave contour that will best reconstruct the contours of the orbital floor, zygoma, and maxilla.

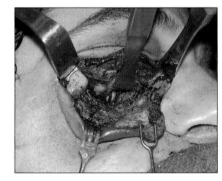

Fig 5-3e Recipient tissue bed prepared to receive calvarial bone grafts for reconstruction of the orbital floor, a portion of the zygoma, and the anterior wall of the maxilla via a modified Weber-Ferguson incision.

Midface reconstruction

For reconstruction of the orbital floor, orbital rims, nasal architecture, or anterior maxillary wall, a calvarial bone graft is preferred. Calvarial grafts have similar contours to these areas and undergo less volume reduction upon incorporation into the graft site (Figs 5-3a to 5-3d). The diploic vascular channels in calvarial bone, which are evolutionarily designed to vent heat generated by brain metabolism, allow earlier and more extensive vascular ingrowth. This early revascularization permits greater cellular survival of the graft and hence a bone resorption-remodeling ratio that is closer to 1:1 than other donor sites. This benefit can be enhanced with the use of PRP. As with maxillary reconstruction, the block component of the graft is lag-screwed with a minimum of two screws to the host bone and/or fixated with 2.0-mm plates (Figs 5-3e and 5-3f). It is then supplemented with cancellous marrow that may be obtained from the marrow space between the inner and outer tables. Before the lag screws are tightened, a layer of PRP should be

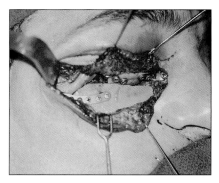

Fig 5-3f Calvarial bone grafts used to reconstruct the orbital floor, zygoma, and anterior wall of the maxilla are fixated with a plate.

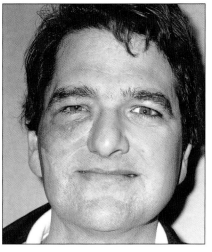

Fig 5-3g Significant improvement in facial contours achieved through calvarial bone grafting.

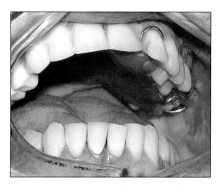

Fig 5-3h Hemi-maxillectomy defect is further rehabilitated by an obturator-denture prosthesis.

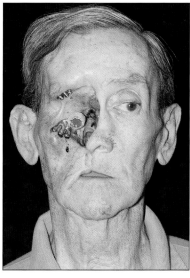

Fig 5-4a Defect of the right orbit, zygoma, maxilla, and a portion of the nose due to basal cell carcinoma and radiotherapy. Bone grafts and dental implants attached to a magnet provide a retentive mechanism for a facial prosthesis.

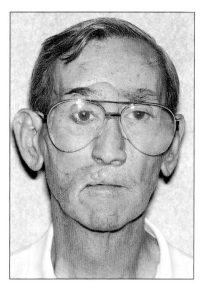

Fig 5-4b Facial prosthesis replacing the right eye and portions of the right cheek and nose allowed this individual to be an active member of society.

placed between the host bone surface and the calvarial graft to accelerate and ensure their union. Several layers of PRP are added to the surface of the graft once it is fixed in place. The outcome is a firm bony reconstruction that should not change in dimension over time and thus will be capable of maintaining increased facial contours (Figs 5-3g and 5-3h) and also capable of supporting external implants for an eye, ear, or nose prosthesis (Figs 5-4a and 5-4b) if needed.

Alveolar Cleft Grafting

Grafting of the nasoalveolar cleft in cleft palate individuals is usually recommended between the ages of 5 and 11 years.[8] Most surgeries in this age group do not require PRP because children heal primarily by cellular regeneration, and their baseline population of healing-capable stem cells is much greater than that of adults.[9] Therefore, upregulating the initial proliferation of the stem cell population and enhancing capillary ingrowth is almost always unnecessary. However, surgery for grafting and closure of an alveolar cleft is the exception. Cleft lip closure is usually accomplished within 3 months of birth, and cleft palate closure usually just before age 3. These surgeries induce significant scar tissue formation and greatly reduce the baseline stem cell population by as early as 5 years. In addition, by age 5, many of these individuals have undergone revisional surgeries or tooth removals, further compromising the potential recipient tissue in the alveolar cleft. To further complicate potential reconstruction, many individuals do not have access to providers of reconstructive and dental procedures until they are well into their teenage years or even into their 20s and 30s. In every age-related study performed to date, the incidence of wound dehiscence, graft infection, graft loss, and redevelopment of the oronasal fistula proportionally increased with age.[10,11] Because of these potential complications, as well as the necessity of closing the fistula and developing a sufficient volume of bone in the cleft for arch integrity, future orthognathic surgery, and dental rehabilitation, PRP is of great value.

Preoperative considerations

The goals of alveolar cleft grafting are *(1)* to stabilize the maxillary arch, *(2)* to develop bone support for canine eruption or dental implant placement, *(3)* to close the oronasal fistulae, and *(4)* to develop bone support for the central incisor and the ala of the nose. It is best to accomplish alveolar cleft grafting at age 5 or 6, if possible, when the risks of complications and graft failure are low and ideal bone support for the central incisor and canine can be developed before they erupt. Grafting accomplished at older ages may be compromised by exposure of cementum into the cleft from the central incisor or canine. In such cases, the amount of bone height that can be gained will be limited to the apical level of the exposed cementum.[12] Attempts to graft to a normal crestal bone height in these cases invite dehiscence and periodontal defects and occasionally even root resorption.[13]

If a lateral incisor remains in the defect, it is best to remove it prior to alveolar cleft grafting. Residual follicular or granulation tissue around this tooth may complicate the graft itself or its soft tissue closure (Fig 5-5a). If the arch is collapsed, as would be expected, it is best to accomplish orthodontic arch expansion before grafting (Fig 5-5b). Although this will increase the size of the defect and the fistula, it will afford more direct access to and visualization of the defect for the all-important nasal floor suturing, and it will increase the amount of soft tissue available for this closure (see Fig 5-5a). The increased amount of bone grafting material needed for this slightly larger defect is insignificant.

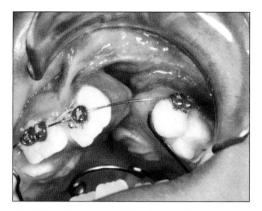

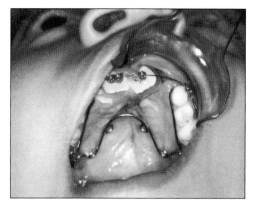

Fig 5-5a Removal of the lateral incisor and any granulation tissue will result in a well-epithelialized and mature fistula amenable to alveolar cleft grafting. (Figs 5-5a and 5-5b are courtesy of Drs Stephen Buckley and Robert P. Johnson, San Antonio, Texas.)

Fig 5-5b Orthodontic arch expansion should be accomplished prior to grafting of the alveolar cleft.

Bone grafting procedure

Despite some authors' suggestions to use allogeneic cancellous bone[14] or autogenous bone from the chin[15] or cranium,[16] autogenous cancellous marrow from the ilium[17] remains the gold standard for grafting alveolar clefts. Its track record of success is unmatched by any other donor site because it provides bone-regenerating endosteal osteoblasts and marrow stem cells. Bone grafting studies using autogenous cancellous marrow from the ilium have shown capillary ingrowth by 5 or 6 days without PRP versus 3 days with PRP and complete revascularization by 20 days without PRP versus 14 days with PRP.[18,19]

The procedure for preparation of the recipient tissue site is essentially identical for unilateral and bilateral clefts, with only minor variations as noted. For both types of clefts, labial and palatal flaps must be fully developed for access to the nasal floor as well as to advance the mucosa to cover the graft. Because of the obvious nasal communication before and during the surgery, intraoperative and postoperative antibiotic coverage for staphylococcal organisms is recommended. Potent antibiotics such as vancomycin, Zyvox (Pharmacia), several cephalosporins, Bactrim (Roche), and Vibramycin (Pfizer US) are most effective.

Incisions are made in the mucogingival area posterior to the cleft with a vertical releasing incision in the second molar area for a sliding labial advancement flap. This incision is carried around the erupted tooth just posterior to the cleft and extended along the palatal gingiva. A similar incision is made anterior to the cleft in the area of the incisors and canine posterior at least to the first premolar area in unilateral clefts (Fig 5-6). In bilateral clefts, the incision anterior to the clefts needs to be carried only to the midpoint of the ipsilateral central incisor because an identical incision will be required on the opposite side. This will maintain a midline labial vascular pedicle to the free-floating pre-maxilla (Fig 5-7a). A vertical incision is then made into the cleft(s) from the marginal gingiva around the tooth

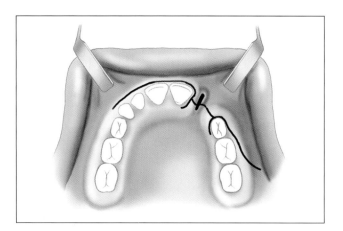

Fig 5-6 Incision placement for a unilateral alveolar cleft graft.

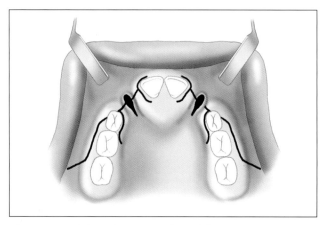

Fig 5-7a Incision placement for a bilateral alveolar cleft graft.

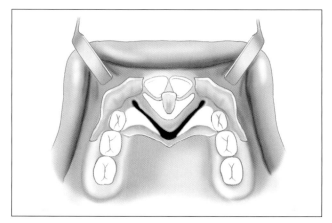

Fig 5-7b Alveolar cleft grafts require thorough reflection of the labial and palatal periosteum to access the nasal floor and achieve a primary closure over the graft with minimal tension.

on each side of the cleft(s). This permits the development of broad-based labial and palatal flaps as well as direct visualization of the nasal floor (Fig 5-7b). Thoroughly reflecting the labial and palatal periosteum and the periosteum of the nasal floor will allow for primary closure of the nasal floor, usually with a 4-0 resorbable suture (Figs 5-8, 5-9a, and 5-9b). Since the tenuous nasal floor closure is critical to the success of the graft, the authors coat the nasal floor with activated PRP (Figs 5-10a to 5-10c) and incubate the graft material in activated PRP for at least 10 minutes before placing it (Fig 5-11). This helps seal the nasal floor and promotes rapid healing without breakdown. It also adds texture to the graft to aid in its placement into the defect and provides the growth factors that promote early revascularization and more complete bone regeneration via the mechanism detailed in chapter 1. The labial and palatal closures must avoid adding tension to the wound. A posterior labial releasing incision allows forward advancement of this tissue, which can be made easier by scoring the periosteum and undermining the tissue (Figs 5-12a and 5-12b). A horizontal or vertical mattress type of everted closure is recommended. The authors also place activated

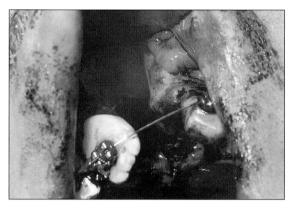

Fig 5-8 Unilateral alveolar cleft with closure of the nasal floor. (Figs 5-8 to 5-15 are courtesy of Drs Stephen Buckley and Robert P. Johnson, San Antonio, Texas.)

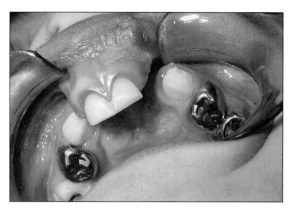

Fig 5-9a Bilateral alveolar clefts with floating pre-maxillary component.

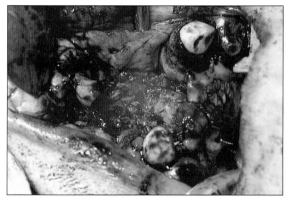

Fig 5-9b The pre-maxillary component in a bilateral alveolar cleft remains pedicled on its labial blood supply as the nasal floor is closed.

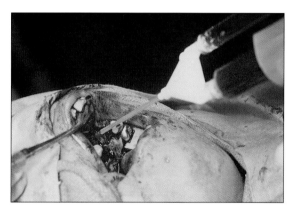

Fig 5-10a The ejection assembly is convenient for coating the nasal floor with PRP.

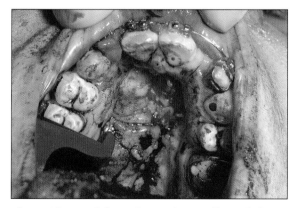

Fig 5-10b Nasal floor closure in a unilateral alveolar cleft.

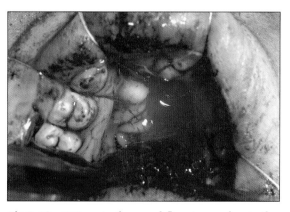

Fig 5-10c PRP coats the nasal floor to accelerate the healing and closure of this critical area.

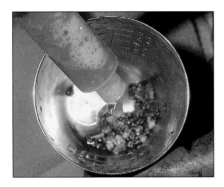

Fig 5-11 An alveolar cleft graft is often incubated in PRP to improve its handling properties and begin its acceleration of osteoprogenitor cell replication.

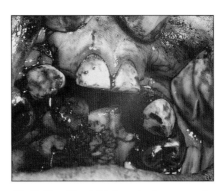

Fig 5-12a The labial periosteum needs to be incised and the labial mucosa undermined to gain a tension-free closure.

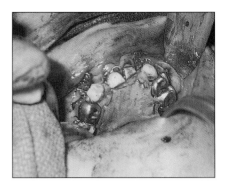

Fig 5-12b A complete tension-free closure of the labial mucosa to the palatal mucosa with eversion of the edges is recommended.

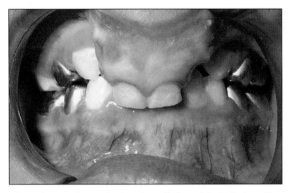

Fig 5-13a Bilateral alveolar clefts with inferior displacement of the pre-maxillary segment.

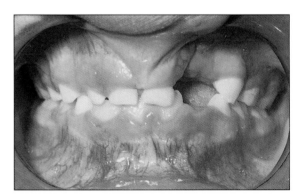

Fig 5-13b After alveolar cleft grafting and repositioning of the pre-maxilla, a normal arch form is created, which can be further rehabilitated with dental implants or other restorative dental procedures.

PRP on the graft surface and on the undersurfaces of each flap, thus virtually eliminating even minor dehiscences and the extrusion of small graft particles (Figs 5-13a and 5-13b) that are common in cases where PRP is not used.

The outcome of alveolar cleft grafting should permit refinement orthodontic therapy and orthognathic surgery. The graft in the defect can be expected to respond to orthodontic as well as orthopedic guidance (ie, distraction devices [Figs 5-14a to 5-14g]) and to accommodate dental implant placement (Figs 5-15a to 5-15d). As the maxilla grows or is guided by orthodontic or orthopedic forces, the bone graft will resorb and remodel with a net gain of bone content to accommodate the growth and expansion in the same manner as native bone grows. The force that can be expected to limit growth and response to orthopedic guidance is the restriction of the soft tissue envelope due to scarring.

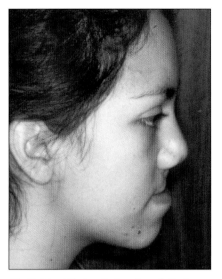

Fig 5-14a Bilateral alveolar clefts have produced a severe anteroposterior maxillary deficiency.

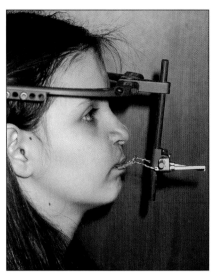

Fig 5-14b Distraction device (KLS Martin) in place. Alveolar cleft grafting will respond to orthodontic treatment, distraction osteogenesis, and maxillary orthognathic surgery.

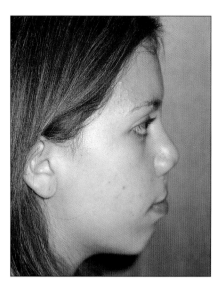

Fig 5-14c Improved facial profile achieved through bilateral alveolar cleft grafting and distraction osteogenesis.

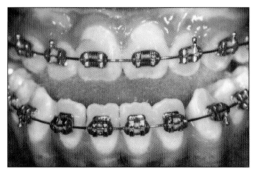

Fig 5-14d Severe Class III malocclusion due to anteroposterior maxillary deficiency in the patient shown in Fig 5-14a following bilateral alveolar cleft grafting.

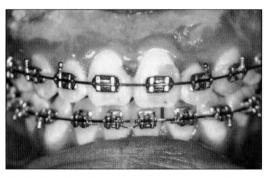

Fig 5-14e Significant improvement to a Class I occlusion with normal overbite and overjet achieved through distraction osteogenesis and orthodontic arch alignment following bilateral cleft grafting.

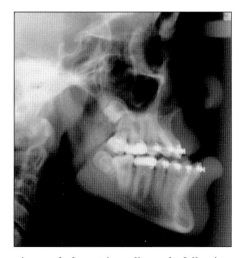

Fig 5-14f Preoperative cephalometric radiograph following bilateral alveolar cleft grafting but prior to distraction osteogenesis showing severe anteroposterior deficiency.

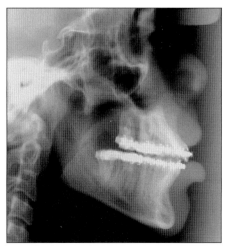

Fig 5-14g Postdistraction cephalometric radiograph showing normal maxillomandibular relationship and normalization of the soft tissue profile.

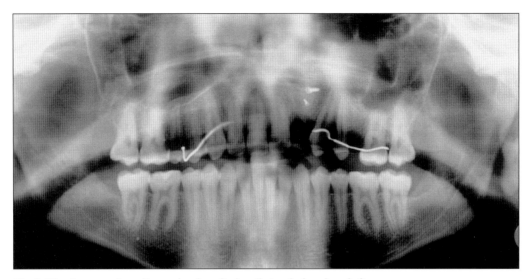

Fig 5-15a Panoramic radiograph of grafted unilateral alveolar cleft.

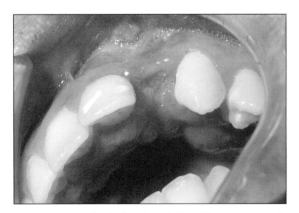

Fig 5-15b Grafted alveolar cleft with normal arch form and spacing for a dental implant to replace the lateral incisor.

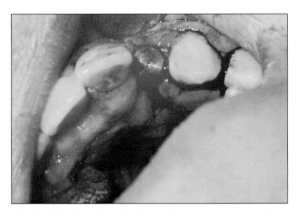

Fig 5-15c Alveolar cleft grafts can accommodate dental implants to restore the lateral incisor or other teeth lost because of the cleft.

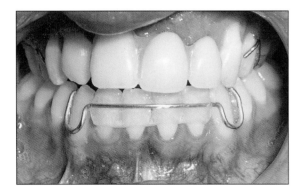

Fig 5-15d Implant-supported restoration of lateral incisor.

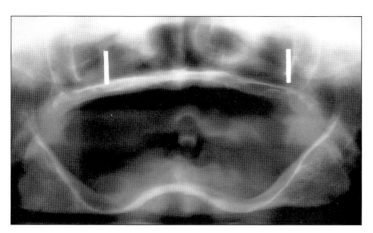

Fig 5-16a Severely resorbed mandible with a maximum height of 4 mm.

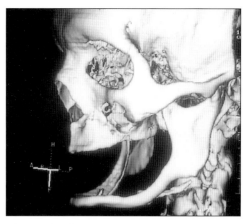

Fig 5-16b The resorbed mandible represents the remnant of the inferior border, which is dense cortical bone. Note that the mandibular canal is unroofed by the resorption process so that the mental nerve now emerges in the second molar region.

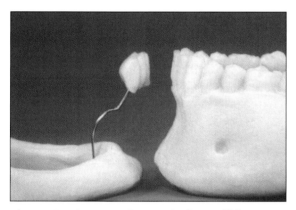

Fig 5-16c The severely resorbed mandible represents a significant and yet often underappreciated loss of vertical bone height.

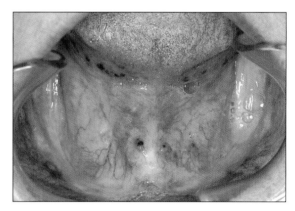

Fig 5-17 The soft tissue mucosa over a severely resorbed mandible is scarred and contracted, indicating a concomitant soft tissue deficiency.

Reconstruction of the Severely Resorbed Mandible

Bony reconstruction, or any surgery involving the severely resorbed mandible, is a strong indication for PRP. A mandible that has resorbed to 6 mm or less at its thinnest point is a common finding in individuals who lost their teeth early in life and have repetitively damaged their mandible and its overlying soft tissue with the compressive forces of denture function or mastication on the edentulous ridge. The residual mandible in these individuals is composed of dense cortical bone, representing the remnant of the inferior border (Figs 5-16a to 5-16c), which is covered by scarred and contracted soft tissue mucosa (Figs 5-17). Adding

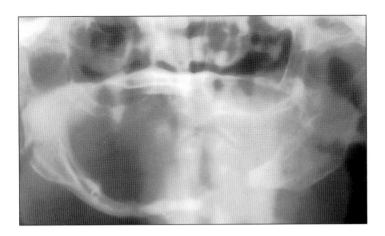

Fig 5-18 Pathologic fractures may occur spontaneously; this one is the result of minor trauma.

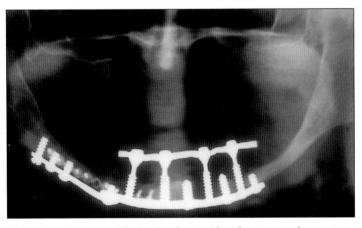

Fig 5-19a Transmandibular implant with a fracture and an extension plate that was placed in an attempt to reduce the fracture. Note the bone resorption around most of the screws and the location of the posteriormost extension plate screw in the mandibular canal.

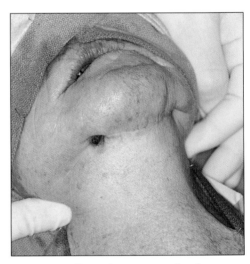

Fig 5-19b Bilateral cutaneous fistulae associated with an infection from a transmandibular implant.

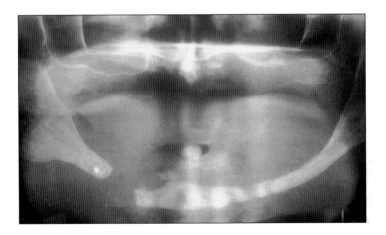

Fig 5-19c Removing a transmandibular implant from a severely resorbed mandible often results in nonvital bone and/or a continuity defect.

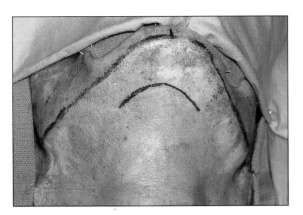

Fig 5-20 Reconstruction of the severely resorbed mandible is approached through a curvilinear incision in the submental triangle.

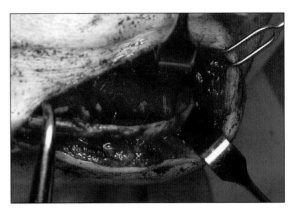

Fig 5-21 The periosteum is reflected from the labial and crestal areas bilaterally to the retromolar areas. In this 4-mm mandible, the left mental nerve emerges from the resorbed crestal bone and the hypertrophied genial tubercles are noted in the midline.

to this problem, 95% of this patient population consists of postmenopausal women with hormone-related osteoporosis. A mandible that has resorbed to 6 mm or less has been known to fracture spontaneously or in response to slight trauma, creating the risk of an airway compromise and usually resulting in a nonunion (Fig 5-18). Before the soft tissue matrix expansion ("tent pole") graft was introduced,[20] grafts for these patients met with myriad healing-related complications and significant resorption of the grafts within 18 months. Alternative reconstructive approaches using prosthetic devices such as the transmandibular implant or the mandibular staple implant have been grossly ineffectual and are themselves associated with a high complication rate from infections, fistulae, and fractures (Figs 5-19a to 5-19c).[20,21] Today, these complications can be avoided and the resorbed mandible predictably reconstructed to 15 mm of height using dental implants to control the soft tissue matrix and PRP to promote rapid bone regeneration in this compromised and elderly patient population.

In this procedure, the mandible is exposed through a curvilinear incision in the submental triangle (Fig 5-20). The incision is centered at the midline 2 cm below the inferior border and extended laterally to a line drawn vertically from each commissure. The soft tissue dissection approaches the mandible at the labial edge, where the periosteum is incised along the length of the incision. Periosteum (and mucosa) is thoroughly reflected from only the crestal and lateral aspects of the mandible. Care is taken to keep the inferior border and lingual periosteum intact to avoid disruption of their blood supply. The mucoperiosteal reflection must extend posteriorly to the masseter on the lateral aspect and past the retromolar trigone and actually up the anterior ramus crestally (Fig 5-21). This creates a volume space for the bone graft. If this volume space is not maintained, it will collapse and contract around the graft, leading to resorption due to natural bone remodeling within 18 months. To avoid this, dental implants are placed from this extraoral approach to "tent pole" the mucosa and keep it elevated. In this way, the surgery expands the soft tissue matrix of the graft, which is maintained by the

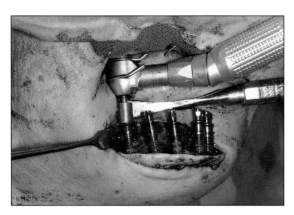

Fig 5-22 The first dental implant is placed 5 mm anterior to the emergence of the mental nerve, and each succeeding implant is placed parallel to and 1 cm apart from center to center.

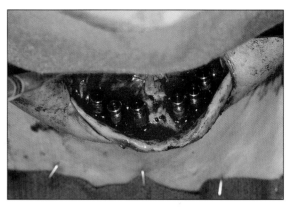

Fig 5-23 The implants gain primary stability by their placement into the inferior border within the buccolingual center of the mandible.

dental implants and is later enhanced by the functional load stimulation generated by an implant-supported prosthesis.

Once the soft tissue has been reflected, 4 to 6 implants are placed into the dense bone of the resorbed mandible. The first implant is positioned 5 mm anterior to the crestal emergence of the inferior alveolar nerve on each side (Fig 5-22), and additional implants are then placed 1 cm apart between these two new mental foramina (Fig 5-23). Each implant should be 15 mm in length and stabilized into or slightly through the inferior border. Thus, in a mandible that has 4 mm of residual height, the implant cover screw extends 11 mm above the bone surface. These 4 to 6 implants will tent the mucosa from their anterior position all the way posterior to the retromolar trigone area.

Once the graft recipient site has been prepared in this fashion, compacted autogenous cancellous marrow, harvested from either the anterior or the posterior ilium, is sequentially placed. The cancellous marrow is placed into a 3- or 5-mL syringe and then compacted by compressing the plunger. The tip of the syringe is then cut so that the graft material can be ejected into each of the four quadrants, starting with the posterior quadrant on each side (Fig 5-24). As the anterior quadrants are grafted, the cancellous marrow must be compacted lingual to and between the implants to the height of each implant. It is pointless and even somewhat wasteful to condense the bone graft over the height of the implants; since contraction of the mucosa is prevented only by the rigidity of the implants, the bone graft will resorb and remodel until it reaches the height of the implant. After it has been placed, the graft is compacted even more densely with the use of bone packers and then covered with a layer of activated PRP (Figs 5-25a to 5-25c). Several applications of activated PRP from a 60-mL blood draw are needed to coat the entire graft. Within 5 minutes the PRP will mature, and its adherence of the cancellous marrow particles will permit a sculpting of the graft to achieve a tapered ridge form (Fig 5-25d).

Fig 5-24 Autogenous cancellous marrow is placed and compacted posterior to each mental nerve emergence and into the retromolar area first.

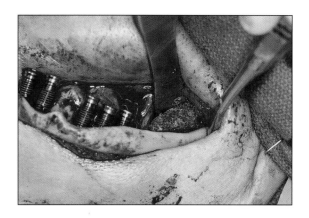

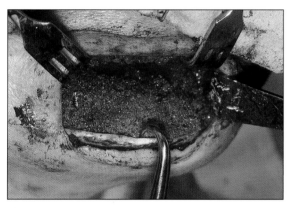

Fig 5-25a Autogenous cancellous marrow is then placed around all of the dental implants and compacted with bone packers to the height of the implant cover screws.

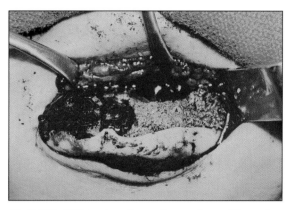

Fig 5-25b PRP is placed over the surface of the autogenous cancellous marrow. Here half of the graft has been covered by PRP, and the other half of the compacted cancellous marrow remains to be covered by PRP.

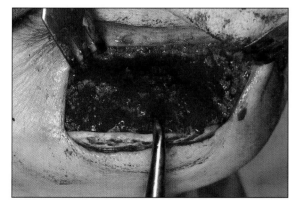

Fig 5-25c The entire graft should be covered with a thick layer of PRP.

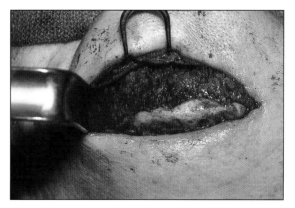

Fig 5-25d Once the PRP covering matures, the clot consistency that it provides allows contouring and sculpting of the graft into a ridge form around the implants.

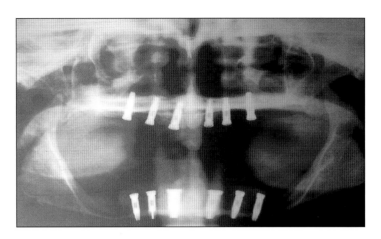

Fig 5-26a Severely resorbed mandible that has been grafted according to the tent-pole procedure, 1 week after surgery. Note the placement of the implants into the inferior border and the absence of mineralization, as one would expect in an autogenous cancellous marrow graft at this time.

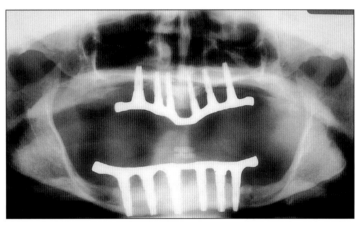

Fig 5-26b Six months after graft placement and 3 months after loading the dental implants with a prosthesis, the mineralization of the graft is more apparent, and 15 mm of bone height have been gained. Note the development of a new mental foramen and mandibular canal in the bone graft.

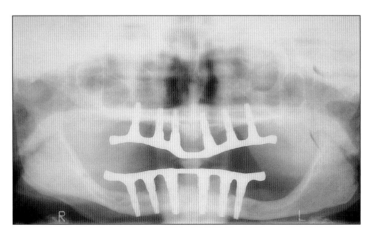

Fig 5-26c Eight-year follow-up of the tent-pole graft attests to the long-term maintenance of the 15-mm bone height, the stability of the implants, and the further mineral density of a graft under functional loading.

The soft tissues are closed without closing the periosteum, which is not only unnecessary given its nonosteogenic quality, but technically impossible due to the expansion of surface area provided by the graft.

Because of such factors as age and osteoporosis, the patients who benefit most from this procedure are also the patients in whom it is most difficult to gain a successful graft. Nonetheless, this procedure has a track record of predictable bone regeneration and permanent maintenance of the original gain in bone height. This is due in part to the support of the graft's soft tissue volume provided by the dental implants, but it is also due to the rapid bone regeneration and maturity

Fig 5-27 The tent-pole grafting procedure provides an ideal bone height, bone density, and contour for denture rehabilitation within a short period of time. Here, permanent dentures were delivered just 4 months after grafting.

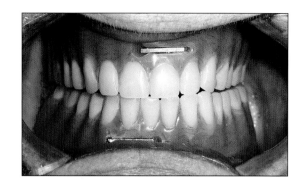

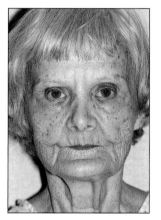

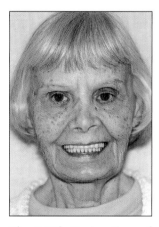

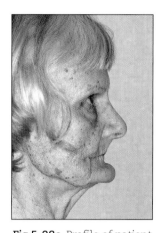

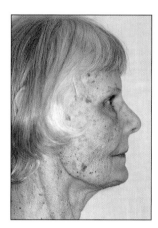

Fig 5-28a Facial collapse due to severely resorbed mandible and maxilla despite the use of dentures.

Fig 5-28b Restoration of facial vertical height and chin contour after tent-pole grafting supported by PRP and new dentures.

Fig 5-28c Profile of patient shown in Fig 5-28a with inadequate dentures in place. Note the loss of facial vertical dimensions and the pointed chin appearance often referred to as the "witch's chin."

Fig 5-28d Correction of facial vertical dimension and a normalized nose-lip-chin relationship and contour as a result of the tent-pole grafting procedure.

gained by the use of PRP. In these cases, the implants are uncovered and functionally loaded at 3 months by the use of a provisional or definitive prosthesis. Because the prosthesis is completely implant-loaded, the functional stresses are transferred to the remodeling bone graft. Once denture loading is achieved, the graft shows a dramatic increase in radiographic density that is maintained permanently (Figs 5-26a to 5-26c).

When PRP is used for this indication, the growth factors and cell adhesion molecules stimulate accelerated bone regeneration and early maturity of bone so that early functional loading can be achieved. This is positive for the graft because it will rapidly increase its density. It is also positive for the patient, who no longer experiences the constant danger of fracturing their mandible and regains the ability to wear a denture that is stable and retentive after just a short healing period (Fig 5-27). Such dramatic results are a testament to what can be achieved using the biology of enhancing bone regeneration together with the engineering mechanics of bone's response to functional stress loading (Figs 5-28a to 5-28d).

References

1. Marx RE, Carlson ER, Eichstaedt RM, Schimmele SR, Strauss JE, Georgeff KR. Platelet-rich plasma: Growth factor enhancement for bone grafts. Oral Surg Oral Med Oral Pathol Oral Radiol Endod 1998;85:638–646.

2. Marx RE. Platelet-rich plasma: Evidence to support its use. J Oral Maxillofac Surg 2004; 62:489–496.

3. Kassolis JD, Rosen PS, Reynolds MA. Alveolar ridge and sinus augmentation utilizing platelet-rich plasma in combination with freeze-dried allograft: Case series. J Periodontol 2000;71:1654–1661.

4. Camargo PM, Lekovic V, Weinlaender M, Vasilic N, Madzarevi M, Kenney EB. Platelet-rich plasma and bovine porous bone mineral combined with guided tissue regeneration in the treatment of intrabony defects in humans. J Periodontal Res 2002;37:300–306.

5. Mancuso J, Bennion JW, Hull MJ, Winterholler BW. Platelet-rich plasma: A preliminary report in routine impacted mandibular third molar surgery and the prevention of alveolar osteitis. J Oral Maxillofac Surg 2003;61(suppl 1).

6. Petrungaro PS. Using platelet-rich plasma to accelerate soft tissue maturation in esthetic periodontal surgery. Compend Contin Educ Dent 2001;22:729–732.

7. Banoth S, Alex JC. Current applications of platelet-gels in plastic surgery. Facial Plast Surg 2002;18:27–32.

8. Boyne PJ, Sands NR. Combined orthodontic-surgical management of residual alveolar cleft defects. Am J Orthod 1976;70:20–37.

9. Caplan AI. Mesenchymal stem cells. J Orthop Res 1991;9:641–650.

10. Bergland O, Semb G, Abyholm F, Borchgrevink H, Eskeland G. Secondary bone grafting and orthodontic treatment in patients with bilateral complete clefts of the lip and palate. Ann Plast Surg 1986;17:460–474.

11. Sindet-Pedersen S, Enemark H. Comparative study of secondary and late secondary bone-grafting in patients with residual cleft defects. Short-term evaluation. Int J Oral Surg 1985;14:389–398.

12. Bergland O, Semb A, Abyholm FE. Elimination of the residual alveolar cleft by secondary bone grafting and subsequent orthodontic treatment. Cleft Palate J 1986;23:175–205.

13. Enemark H, Sindet-Pedersen S, Bundgaard M. Long-term results after secondary bone grafting of alveolar clefts. J Oral Maxillofac Surg 1987;45:913–919.

14. Belts NJ, Fonseca RJ. Allogeneic grafting of dentoalveolar clefts. In: Hudson JW (ed). Oral and Maxillofacial Surgery Clinics of North America—Management of Cleft Lip and Palate. Philadelphia: WB Saunders, 1991:617–624.

15. Sindet-Pedersen S, Enemark H. Reconstruction of alveolar clefts with mandibular or iliac crest bone grafts. A comparison study. J Oral Maxillofac Surg 1990;48:554–558.

16. Wolfe SA, Berkowitz S. The use of cranial bone grafts in the closure of alveolar and anterior palatal clefts. Plast Reconstr Surg 1983;72:659–671.

17. Hall DH, Werther JR. Conventional alveolar cleft bone grafting. In: Hudson JW (ed). Oral and Maxillofacial Surgery Clinics of North America—Management of Cleft Lip and Palate. Philadelphia: WB Saunders, 1991:609–616.

18. Albrektsson T. Repair of bone grafts: A vital microscopic and histologic investigation in the rabbit. Scand J Plast Reconstr Surg 1980;14:1–12.

19. Marx RE. Platelet-rich plasma: A source of multiple autogenous growth factors for bone grafts. In: Lynch SE, Genco RJ, Marx RE (eds). Tissue Engineering. Applications in Maxillofacial Surgery and Periodontics. Chicago: Quintessence, 1999:71–82.

20. Marx RE, Shellenberger T, Wimsatt J, Correa P. Severely resorbed mandible: Predictable reconstruction with soft tissue matrix expansion (tent pole) grafts. J Oral Maxillofac Surg 2002;60:878–888.

21. Betts NJ, Powers M, Barber HD. Reconstruction of the severely atrophic edentulous mandible with the transmandibular implant systems. J Oral Maxillofac Surg 1995;53:295–304.

Soft Tissue Craniofacial Applications

Rhytidectomy

The desire for facial cosmetic surgery in our society continues to grow. Once the exclusive province of Hollywood movie stars and the elite, facial cosmetic surgery is now considered a social and economic necessity by many Americans. Along with the desire for facial improvement, however, comes an expectation for uncomplicated healing and a favorable result. Every surgeon who performs facial cosmetic surgery tries to understand the patient's expectations and to communicate the limitations of cosmetic surgery. Despite receiving adequate forewarning and providing informed consent, however, patients often expect a perfect result as well as a postoperative course that is free of complications.

The most common complication of a rhytidectomy, or face lift surgery, is ecchymosis (bruising), which itself is not serious and can be expected to resolve spontaneously. However, it almost always disappoints the patient and delays his or her return to the workplace and normal activities. Ecchymosis may also progress into a hematoma and/or an infection, both of which pose a risk of skin slough (Fig 6-1), by far the most dreaded complication in a face lift surgery. Therefore, hemostasis is critical to achieving a result that is free of complications and avoiding a result that is potentially disastrous. Hematomas will raise and distend the skin flap from the deep tissue base. The tension created by the hematoma will inhibit venous drainage and then capillary fill of the skin flap. The skin will become shiny and start peeling, and necrosis will cause it to turn black. A hematoma requires prompt drainage so as to prevent skin necrosis, but it will nevertheless

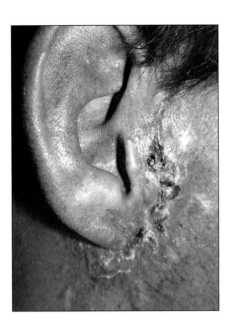

Fig 6-1 Wound dehiscence and infection significantly compromised the outcome of this rhytidectomy.

compromise the cosmetic result. Therefore, absolute hemostasis and prevention of a hematoma are crucial. The hemostatic properties of platelet-rich plasma (PRP) and platelet-poor plasma (PPP) promote a state of absolute hemostasis and thereby prevent ecchymosis and the formation of a hematoma. Collapse of the dead space beneath the flap as a result of adherence by the cell adhesion molecules in PRP and PPP also increases resistance to hematoma formation and infection.

After skin slough, the most dreaded complication related to wound healing is flap dehiscence and excessive scarring. In the nonkeloid patient, these complications occur as a result of closure under tension and are therefore more common in the postauricular area. Adler and Kent have shown that closure under mild tension, which is very common, is associated with reduced scar formation and an absence of wound dehiscence when PRP is used (Figs 6-2a and 6-2b).[1] The benefits of PRP's hemostatic properties have also been demonstrated by Adler, who routinely accomplishes face lifts without the use of drains (Figs 6-2c to 6-2e).[1] In addition to faster healing at the flap incision line, PRP can limit or reduce the amount of hair loss associated with face lift surgery. In the temporal and postauricular areas, minor but detracting hair loss along the incision line can result from damage to the local blood supply at the flap margin and hence to the cells in the hair follicle. In most cases the hair follicle recovers and slowly regenerates over the next 3 to 6 months. However, in some cases the hair fails to regenerate, leaving an unsightly band of alopecia that betrays the fact that the individual has recently undergone cosmetic surgery (Fig 6-3). The growth factors in PRP reduce or prevent such hair loss by stimulating capillary ingrowth so that the compromised cells of the hair follicle survive and regenerate hair more quickly.

Other known complications of face lift surgery, such as facial nerve injury, earlobe distortion (the so-called bat wing deformity), and other causes of skin slough, arise from technical problems that PRP cannot prevent. It is even more important in discussing PRP's role in facial cosmetic surgery to remind the surgeon that PRP is an adjunct to and not a substitute for precise surgery.

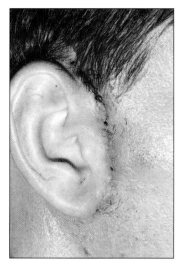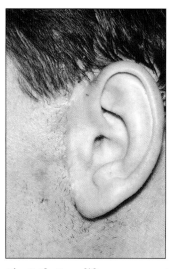

Fig 6-2a Face lift surgery, postoperative day 7. Right-side incision was closed with fast-absorbing catgut sutures. Note the erythema and friable skin edges. (Figs 6-2a to 6-2e courtesy of Dr Stephen Adler, Stuart, Florida.)

Fig 6-2b Face lift surgery, postoperative day 7. Left-side incision of same patient was closed with PRP and without cutaneous sutures. Note the reduced degree of inflammation, erythema, and swelling and the more rapid epithelialization compared with Fig 6-2a.

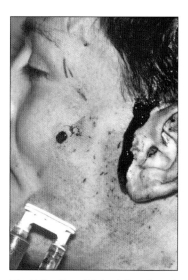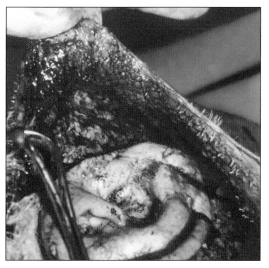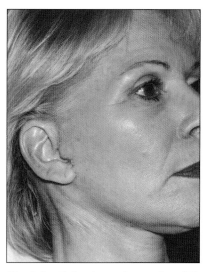

Fig 6-2c Face lift incision closed with deep 5-0 polydioxane sutures and tension-free cutaneous sutures with PRP. Note the droplet of coagulated PRP on the cheek.

Fig 6-2d The side that received PRP shows a septated bridging coagulum attaching the undersurface of the flap to the deep soft tissue surface. This is the result of the cell adhesion molecules in PRP, which eliminate dead space within the flap.

Fig 6-2e Eight days after a face lift surgery using PRP, this patient showed minimal edema and no ecchymosis.

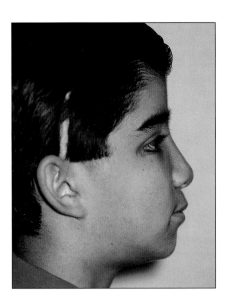

Fig 6-3 Alopecia due to hair follicle loss from incision line dehiscence and delayed healing.

The placement of incisions and the surgical techniques used in face lift surgery have numerous variations, as the literature amply demonstrates, but they all share certain basic principles. Most face lift surgeries call for a curvilinear incision in the temporal skin, which extends vertically into the preauricular skin fold and then curves into the postauricular area below the ear lobule (Fig 6-4). Care should be taken to avoid the hair-bearing area of the sideburns. By beveling the incision in the hair-bearing areas of the temporal region, disturbance of the blood supply to the hair follicles, and thus the potential for hair loss, is minimized. The skin is then undermined at a plane deep to the superficial musculoaponeurotic system (SMAS), which is a cutaneous fascial layer that includes the superficial temporal fascia and its extension over the parotid gland, the cheek, and the superficial surface of the platysma muscle.[2]

A two-part flap is created. The preauricular portion of the flap is intended to elevate the cheek and eliminate the jowls. The postauricular portion is intended to elevate the neck and tighten the submental area. Each skin flap is undermined approximately 5 to 6 cm using Reese face lift scissors, which have dual cutting edges. An even thickness of the skin-SMAS level is obtained when the scissors are advanced in the dissection in the closed position and then gently opened as they are withdrawn. The skin flaps are then pulled to assess the desired lift, and the excess skin is excised.[3] If there are any bleeding vessels remaining in the wound, they should be cauterized. Prior to closing, 4 to 5 mL of PRP should be applied to the undermined skin flap and along the edges of the flap (Fig 6-5).

As noted earlier, the fibrin-fibronectin-vitronectin cell adhesion molecules in the PRP will promote absolute hemostasis, a critical factor in the avoidance of ecchymosis and the formation of a hematoma, which is an even more worrisome sign.[4] The PRP also helps the skin-SMAS flaps adhere to the deeper fascia and hence reduce the amount of dead space (see Fig 6-2d). The seven growth factors contained in PRP will accelerate capillary, collagen, and nerve ingrowth from the

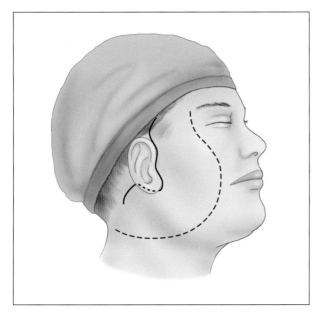

Fig 6-4 Standard rhytidectomy incision with undermined area of skin and SMAS layer. The deep tissue base and undersurface of the skin-SMAS layer are extensive surface areas to be healed.

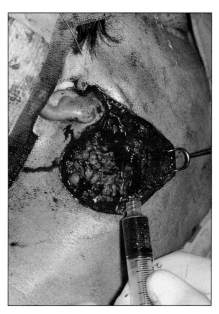

Fig 6-5 Activated PRP should be applied to the undersurface of the skin-SMAS flap and along the edges of the skin incision.

deeper fascia to the skin flaps and across the incision lines to reduce scarring and limit hair follicle loss. Eliminating dead space and speeding up regeneration of the blood supply also promotes healing indirectly by reducing the potential for bacterial infections and for viral eruptions of the skin. The use of PRP can also be expected to accelerate the rate and degree of skin sensation return.[5] The development of skin flaps itself severs small sensory nerve fibers to the skin, and although it usually abates within 3 to 6 months, this sensory loss is of great concern to the patient, and in some cases it may never normalize completely. PRP is theorized to accelerate the return of skin sensation via its growth factor stimulation of capillary ingrowth and collagen synthesis, which support nerve regeneration.[6]

Additional PRP may be used if more hemostasis is needed or if the tissue flap requires greater adherence. Otherwise, traction sutures are used to suspend the SMAS to the temporal and mastoid areas for the desired degree of facial tightening. This is followed by a subcuticular and skin closure to maintain even positioning of the skin flap. At the start of the subcuticular closure, a small amount of PRP can be added along the incision line if necessary.

Face lift surgery requires application of a Barton type of pressure dressing, which should remain in place for 2 to 3 days, followed by ice for 48 hours, elevation of the head, and the use of hydrogen peroxide/antibiotic ointment to promote healing of the incision area.

Blepharoplasty

After face lift surgery, the most common facial cosmetic surgery is blepharoplasty, which is designed to correct baggy eyelids by excising redundant skin and muscle. With blepharoplasties, as with face lift surgery, a less-than-perfect result is tantamount to a poor result; potential side effects include excessive tearing, xerophthalmia, excessive scleral show, conjunctivitis, ectropion (eversion of the eyelid), and even entropion (inversion of the eyelid), with or without eyelash injury to the cornea (known as *trichiasis*). The success of a blepharoplasty procedure hinges on a correct assessment of the problem (ie, skin, muscle, fat, or a combination of these), a precisely controlled surgical technique, and rapid, uncomplicated healing. The role of PRP in a blepharoplasty, as in a face lift, is to accelerate the rate and reduce the complications of healing.

Upper eyelid blepharoplasty

With the patient seated and eyes in the relaxed forward gaze, a skin marker is used to mark the curvature of the redundant skin fold, approximately 7 to 10 mm above the ciliary margin. Medially, this line ends just superior to the punctum, while laterally it extends along and above the tarsal plate, ending in or parallel to a natural lateral crease approximately 1 cm lateral to the lateral canthus. A second line is drawn superior and parallel to the first line and blended into it medially and laterally. The width of the area between the lines represents the amount of redundant tissue (Fig 6-6a). To determine how much of this redundant tissue to excise, a tissue forceps is used to grasp the tissue just until it begins to produce a lagophthalmos, at the same time taking care to leave sufficient eyelid skin below the eyebrow so that when the skin edges are approximated, the eyebrow is not inferiorly displaced.

Incisions are made precisely along these planned lines. The redundant skin is excised first in order to expose the fibers of the orbicularis oculi (Fig 6-6b). Next, the amount of redundant muscle to be excised is determined by having the patient open and close the eyes several times. Rarely is there a need to excise as much muscle as skin. The redundant muscle to be excised will appear as a rolled strip and is excised just superior to the tarsal plate and along the entire length of the incision.

Removal of the redundant muscle will expose some of the orbital fat. How much fat to remove is usually estimated preoperatively, but placing light pressure on the globe will cause any excess fat to protrude and allow the surgeon to confirm the estimate during the time of surgery. The excess fat is sharply excised using minimal retraction. Aggressive retraction of the fat often leads the surgeon to excise more fat than intended and results in an irregularly excised edge. The resultant wound includes exposed orbital fat, muscle, and the skin edges. A 1.5-mL volume of activated PRP developed from a 20-mL draw of autologous blood is applied to the surgical site (Fig 6-6c). The value of PRP in blepharoplasty surgery is similar to that in face lift surgery. The adherence properties of PRP and PPP eliminate dead space and will complement the simple surface closure with a 6-0 nonresorb-

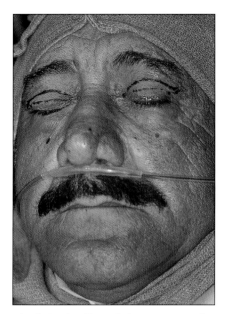

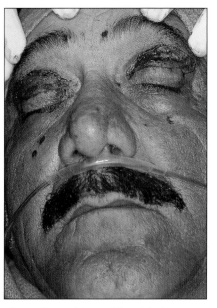

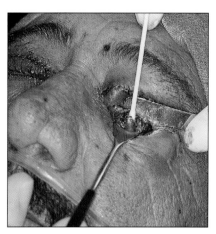

Fig 6-6a Outline of tissue composite to be excised for an upper eyelid blepharoplasty. (Figs 6-6a to 6-6e courtesy of Dr Mark R. Stevens, Miami, Florida.)

Fig 6-6b Excision of the skin between the two marked incision lines will expose a portion of the orbicularis oculi. Any redundant muscle and a small amount of fat are then excised, creating a tissue area onto which the PRP is placed.

Fig 6-6c Activated PRP is applied directly to the blepharoplasty wound prior to closure.

able suture. The hemostatic properties of PRP and PPP reduce the ecchymosis that can result in a so-called raccoon-eye appearance, excessive scarring, and, ultimately, lid retraction. The seven growth factors in PRP accelerate healing to minimize scarring.

Lower eyelid blepharoplasty

Lower eyelid blepharoplasty is less forgiving than upper eyelid blepharoplasty and has more potential for complications.[7] The position of the lower lid and the effects of gravity make lower lid blepharoplasties more likely to result in eyelid laxity, excessive scleral show, and ectropion. Any imperfection in the assessment of the problem, the surgical technique, or wound healing will have a more significant impact on the outcome.

As described above for upper eyelid blepharoplasty, the lower eyelid is marked while the patient is in a seated, relaxed position looking forward. The first line is drawn parallel to and approximately 2 to 3 mm below the ciliary margin. This line should begin just below and lateral to the punctum of the inferior canaliculus and extend laterally beyond the lateral canthus into a natural crease. At the lateral one third of the lid, it should gradually diverge an additional 1 mm below the ciliary margin before blending into a natural lateral crease. An inferior-based skin flap is

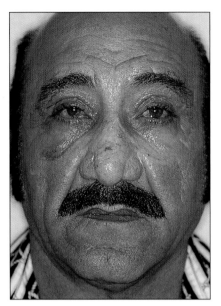

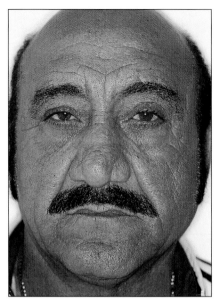

Fig 6-6d Appearance of patient before upper and lower eyelid blepharoplasties using PRP.

Fig 6-6e Elimination of the baggy eyelid appearance and a more alert expression after blepharoplasties using PRP to enhance healing.

then developed via dissection superficial to the orbicularis oculi. As in the upper eyelid blepharoplasty, the patient should open and close the eye so that the surgeon can determine the amount of redundant muscle to excise. Following the fiber direction of the muscle, a strip of muscle is excised, but a rim of pretarsal muscle is preserved to maintain the muscle's function. The amount of excess orbital fat can now be assessed based on the preoperative evaluation and on the amount of fat that protrudes when slight digital pressure is placed on the globe. (The excised fat often can be used in the adjacent areas of skin depression and therefore should not be discarded. As described in the following section, PRP can be used to enhance the survival of these small fat grafts without delayed shrinkage.) After the excess fat and muscle have been excised, the skin flap is approximated to the subciliary incision line. The excess skin is excised, and the skin flap is draped passively over the excised wound to prevent closure with an inferior traction vector, which will result in an excessive scleral show and/or an ectropion. A 1.5-mL volume of activated PRP is applied to each eyelid surgical site at this time and the skin flap closed using a 6-0 nonresorbable suture. Since blepharoplasties are not conducive to postoperative pressure dressings, the hemostatic and adherence properties of PRP are an even stronger consideration in this procedure than they are in face lifts. The enhancement and acceleration of healing should reduce ecchymosis and the potential for healing complications and will result in less overall scarring (Figs 6-6d and 6-6e), as has been shown in skin graft healing and observed in face lift outcomes.

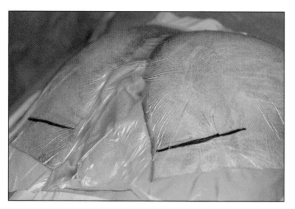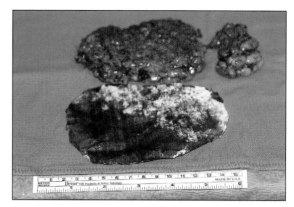

Figs 6-7a and 6-7b The gluteal crease is a convenient and cosmetic site for harvesting a measurable amount of dermal fat.

Dermal Fat Grafts

The excessive hospital time, morbidity, and unpredictability associated with free vascularized fasciocutaneous flaps have led to renewed interest in the more straightforward free nonvascularized dermal fat grafts for facial augmentation.

Historically, dermal fat grafts were regarded as unpredictable, inadequate in size, and subject to dimensional changes.[8] Dermal fat grafts often developed infections and/or underwent necrosis, especially when large-volume grafts were accomplished. Those that healed without such complications would often shrink in size, thus compromising the result or even necessitating another graft. Efforts to over-contour a dermal fat graft by using 20% to 30% more graft material would often be stymied because some grafts would shrink more than anticipated and some would shrink less.[9] Over time, dermal fat grafts developed a reputation for never being right the first time, and larger defects would be planned for two grafting procedures so as to avoid the necrosis of larger graft volumes.

Today, PRP's pivotal role in dermal fat grafting has prompted a resurgence of interest in its use. As with other applications of PRP, the principles and techniques of harvesting, handling, and placing the graft should not be trivialized. The harvesting of graft material requires an absolute sterile technique and should be limited to areas where fat is naturally found and normally deposited in sufficient or even excessive quantities. The authors use the gluteal crease to harvest subcutaneous fat in thin-bodied individuals (Figs 6-7a and 6-7b) and an abdominal skin fold to harvest extraperitoneal subcutaneous fat in individuals with excess fat (Figs 6-8a and 6-8b). The fat should be removed with minimal trauma and without particulation and placed in saline or nonactivated PRP to prevent dehydration and to maintain lipoblast and lipocyte survival (Fig 6-9). Harvesting of the fat from the donor site should be timed to coincide with the recipient site prepara-

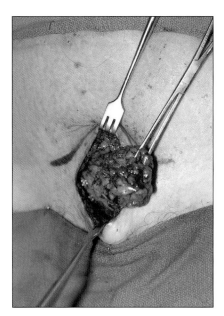

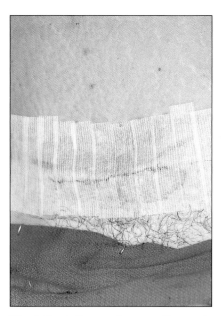

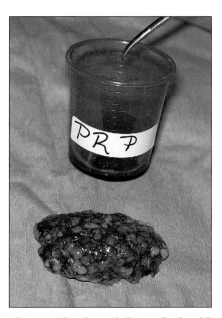

Fig 6-8a A natural fold in the supra-pubic area is another convenient and cosmetic site for harvesting dermal fat.

Fig 6-8b A linear closure of a peri-umbilical or supra-pubic incision can be accomplished with dermal sutures supported by Steri-Strips (3M). The incision will eventually resemble a natural skin crease.

Fig 6-9 The dermal fat graft should not be particulated. Ideally, it should be taken directly from the donor site and placed into the recipient site. If it cannot be placed immediately into the recipient site, incubation in nonactivated PRP or even saline will maintain lipoblast and lipocyte survival.

tion or accomplished by a separate surgical team to minimize the amount of time the graft is outside the body. At the recipient site, the epidermis and full thickness of the dermis should be maintained as a minimum thickness and may include all or a portion of the subcutaneous layer if it is present.

The authors recommend placing activated PRP on the graft prior to placement and then covering it with additional PRP afterward. It would be imprudent to use all of the PRP prior to graft placement because some will be lost or suctioned away as the graft is fitted into the recipient site. For maximum stability, the graft should be sutured to the base of the recipient site. To avoid creating a line of demarcation between the graft and the adjacent native tissue, it is often necessary to taper the edges of the graft and to use external bolsters to develop a gradual blending of the graft to native tissue as well as to stabilize the graft. The bolsters are placed using a 3-0 or 4-0 nylon or prolene suture on a threaded needle, which is passed through the native skin into the recipient wound space. The needle should enter the skin 1 to 2 cm from the edge of the wound space; the needle should enter the actual wound space at the very edge, where the native tissue joins the wound space (Fig 6-10a). The needle is then passed through one edge of the dermal fat graft and out again, engaging a 5- to 8-mm section of the graft in a fashion similar to a horizontal mattress suture. The needle is then passed through the wound space at the point where it adjoins native tissue and out the skin 5 to 8 mm from the needle's entrance point (Fig 6-10b), again similar in concept to a horizontal mattress suture. As the sutures are tightened, the dermal fat

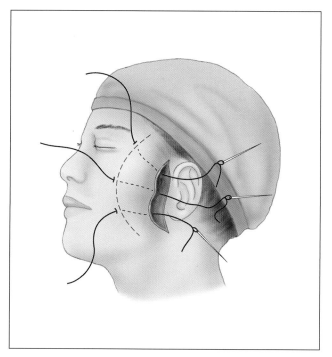

Fig 6-10a Skin flap with nylon sutures placed through the skin into the wound space.

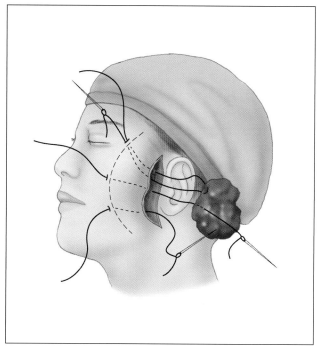

Fig 6-10b The sutures go through the dermal fat graft and exit adjacent to their point of entry after passing back through the wound space.

graft is advanced into the recipient wound space (Figs 6-10c and 6-10d). The sutures are tied to a sterile button, plastic tube, or cotton roll, which can serve as a bolster (Fig 6-10e). This maneuver will allow the surgeon to observe and evaluate the size and shape of the graft and to determine whether to make adjustments before final closure. Once the final contour is attained, about 5 to 10 mL of PRP is added to the surface of the graft and over the entire recipient wound space (Fig 6-10f).

The clinical value of applying PRP during this procedure is enhanced lipoblast and lipocyte survival, and hence dimensional stability. When PRP is used, the surgeon does not need to place an excessive volume of fat in the volume space because there is little or no contraction of the graft and therefore no loss of contour (Figs 6-10g and 6-10h). In addition, surgeons who use PRP have observed a lower incidence of infections and skin dehiscence as well as less swelling and skin bruising.[10] These benefits are related to accelerated capillary ingrowth into the graft, which allows for complete or nearly complete fat cell survival. The problems previously noted to be associated with dermal fat grafts are partly a result of delayed capillary ingrowth, which leads to the death of a large population of lipoblasts and lipocytes. When these fat cells necrose, the problem is compounded because the triglycerides and fatty acids contained within them spill out into the wound space and provoke an intense inflammation. This reaction, in turn, produces swelling, pain, occasional skin dehiscence, and additional fat necrosis. The

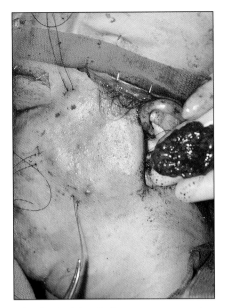

Fig 6-10c The bolster sutures enter and emerge through the dermal fat graft and exit adjacent to their point of entry after passing back through the wound space.

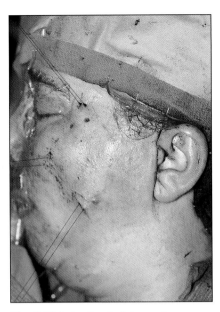

Fig 6-10d As the bolster sutures are tightened, the dermal fat graft is pulled into the wound space and evenly distributed to achieve a gradual tapering of the native tissue and an even placement within the wound space.

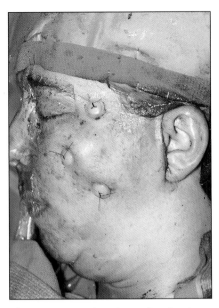

Fig 6-10e Tension is maintained on the sutures for even stability of the dermal fat graft as the sutures are tied to external buttons to resist the pull of gravity.

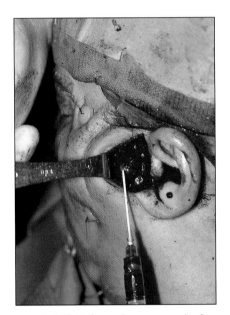

Fig 6-10f Before the pre-auricular incision is closed, activated PRP is placed on the graft and on the incision line closures.

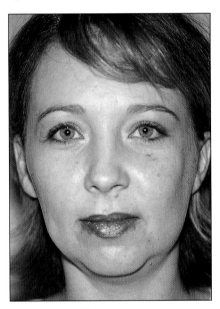

Fig 6-10g Individual with soft tissue cheek deficiency resulting from removal of a tumor.

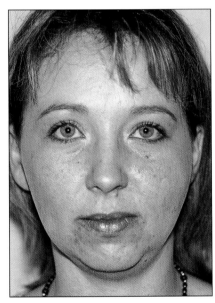

Fig 6-10h The individual shown in Fig 6-10g following dermal fat grafting with PRP as demonstrated in Figs 6-10a through 6-10f.

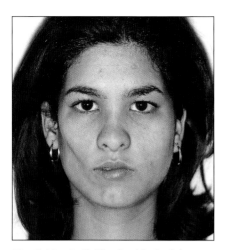

Fig 6-11a Individual with facial atrophy of the right side due to Parry-Romberg syndrome.

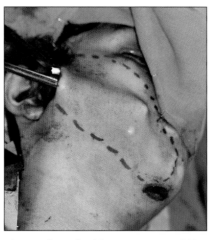

Fig 6-11b A rhytidectomy type of dissection is used to develop recipient tissue for a dermal fat graft.

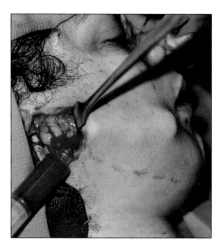

Fig 6-11c Dermal fat graft harvested from the gluteal crease is placed with activated PRP.

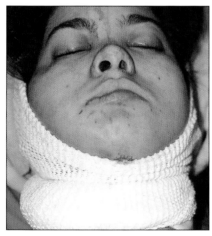

Fig 6-11d When a dermal fat graft is placed, pressure dressings are required to reduce dead space and to stabilize the graft.

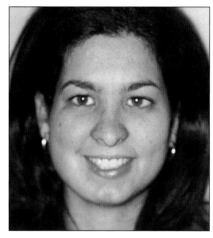

Fig 6-11e Predictable correction of facial atrophy to normal contours is achieved using dermal fat grafting with PRP enhancement.

result is a graft that shrinks to an unpredictable degree and may calcify, develop internal abscesses, and cause unsightly scars. PRP's capacity to promote a rapid capillary ingrowth addresses all of the shortcomings historically associated with dermal fat grafts and has brought the technique back into the mainstream of surgery for facial augmentation as a straightforward procedure associated with reduced morbidity and hospitalization or as an outpatient surgery. Its use can be applied to soft tissue deficiencies from tumor surgery (see Figs 6-10a to 6-10h), trauma, and congenital or developmental defects (Figs 6-11a to 6-11e).

References

1. Adler SC, Kent KJ. Enhancing healing with growth factors. Facial Plast Surg Clin North Am 2002;10:129–146.
2. Mitz V, Peyronie M. The superficial musculo-aponeurotic system (SMAS) in the parotid and cheek area. Plast Reconstr Surg 1976;58:80–88.
3. Alexander RW. Cosmetic alterations of the aging neck. In: Epker BN (ed). Oral and Maxillofacial Surgery Clinics of North America: Cosmetic Oral and Maxillofacial Surgery, vol 2. Philadelphia: WB Saunders, 1990:247–257.
4. Kent KJ. Promising results from a preliminary study of autologous platelet gel in face-lift surgery. Arch Facial Plast Surg 2001;3:251.
5. Welsh W. Autologous platelet gel: Clinical function and useage in plastic surgery. Cosmet Dermatol 2000;13:13–19.
6. Powell DM, Chang E, Farrior EH. Recovery from deep-plane rhytidectomy following unilateral wound treatment with autologous platelet gel: A pilot study. Arch Facial Plast Surg 2001;3:245–250.
7. Kennedy B. Primary blepharoplasty of upper and lower eyelids. In: Epker BN (ed). Oral and Maxillofacial Surgery Clinics of North America: Cosmetic Oral and Maxillofacial Surgery, vol 2. Philadelphia: WB Saunders, 1990:403–412.
8. Niechajev I, Sevcuk O. Long-term results of fat transplantation: Clinical and histologic studies. Plast Reconstr Surg 1994;94:496–506.
9. Pinski KS, Roenigk HH Jr. Autologous fat transplantation: Long-term follow-up. J Dermatol Surg Oncol 1992;18:179–184.
10. Abuzeni PZ, Alexander RW. Enhancement of autologous fat transplantations with platelet-rich plasma. Am J Cosmet Surg 2001;18:59–70.

Phlebotomy Principles/Techniques and PRP Consent Form

At a prestigious international conference on oral surgical and periodontal procedures held in 2004, a prominent and clinically respected periodontist was asked by the moderator why she did not use platelet-rich plasma (PRP). Her candid (and somewhat apologetic) answer was that she did not know how to draw blood. Sterile phlebotomy is a basic technique that is valuable, straightforward, and easy to learn. It is germane not only to the processing of PRP, but also to the administration of antibiotics and of drugs in elective intravenous sedation or potentially life-saving emergency situations. Generations of dental, medical, and nursing students have received training to work as phlebotomists in hospitals in order to cover their tuition and living expenses. There is no reasonable excuse for today's professional healthcare providers to deny their patients the obvious benefits of intravenous access, and now autologous blood components such as PRP, merely because they do not know how to draw blood.

Like any technical dental or medical skill, learning phlebotomy requires didactic education, guided mentorship, and practice. After reading this brief tutorial, the practitioner learning phlebotomy is strongly encouraged to follow up by participating in a phlebotomy workshop or by seeking one-on-one instruction from an experienced clinician combined with repetitive practice. Phlebotomy skills will broaden the practitioner's scope of practice, add an element of safety to all areas of treatment, and enable the practitioner to offer his or her patients access to the growth factors and cell adhesion molecules discussed in this text.

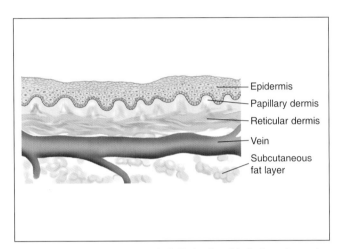

Fig A-1 Veins course superficially in the skin below the reticular dermis and in the uppermost layer of the subcutaneous compartment.

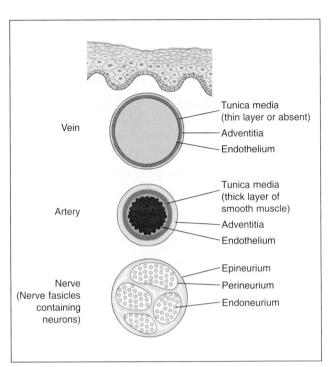

Fig A-2 Veins are anatomically located superficial to arteries, which in turn are superficial to nerves.

Vein and Skin Anatomy

The needle or the plastic catheter used to draw blood and administer medications must pass through skin and the wall of a vein. The skin consists of two layers: the epidermis, which is the epithelium and basement membrane, and the dermis, which consists of the papillary dermis just beneath the basement membrane and around the rete pegs and the larger reticular dermis beneath the papillary dermis and superficial to the subcutaneous layer. The veins that are accessed in phlebotomy course through the subcutaneous layer of the skin (Fig A-1). Nerve fibers, sweat glands, sebaceous glands, and hair follicles traverse the subcutaneous layer into the dermis; hair shafts and sweat glands also pass through the epidermis onto the skin surface. The skin superficial to the vein will therefore be firm and offer some resistance during a venipuncture. As the needle enters the subcutaneous layer, a release of resistance may be felt. Because it is composed mainly of fat, the subcutaneous layer lacks firmness, thus allowing the vein to move or roll if not stabilized by the phlebotomist.

Although veins are known to have thin walls, the walls are composed of three layers: a tunica intima, a tunica media, and a tunica adventitia. Arterial walls are composed of the same three layers, but a thicker basal lamina separates the endothelium of the tunica intima from the tunica media. In addition, the tunica

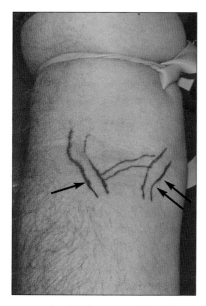

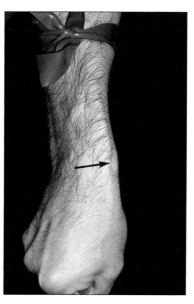

Fig A-3 The common veins in the antecubital fossa that are suitable for phlebotomy and PRP development are the cephalic vein *(arrow)*, the basilic vein *(double arrows)*, and their collateral connecting vein, the median antecubital vein.

Fig A-4 The base of the cephalic vein *(arrow)* is a large stable vein suitable for phlebotomy and PRP development. It is located over the wrist joint proximal to the thumb.

media itself contains many more layers of smooth muscle, adding greater thickness to the wall of the artery (Fig A-2). The venous wall can be entered easily, but it can also be torn easily; when this happens during phlebotomy, it causes the vein to leak (referred to as an "infiltrating" or a "blown" vein) and makes phlebotomy unsuccessful. Unlike arteries, veins have valves that prevent the backflow of blood. If a needle or catheter is inserted into the lumen of a vein and rests against a valve, blood cannot be withdrawn and intravenous solutions will not flow. Repositioning the needle or catheter by rotating it or withdrawing it a short distance can resolve this problem in most cases.

Clinical Vein Identification

Because it is the most stable location from which to draw blood or start an intravenous access, the arm is the site preferred by most clinicians. For drawing blood, it is important to select the largest and most stable vein available. In most cases this will be one of the three more obvious veins in the antecubital fossa: the cephalic vein, the basilic vein, or the median antecubital vein, which is a collateral connection between the cephalic vein and the basilic vein (Fig A-3). Another option is the base of the cephalic vein, which is the large and stable vein located over the wrist joint proximal to the thumb (Fig A-4). In muscular individuals, the cephalic vein is more superficial near the level of the elbow in the antecubital fossa, as is the median antebrachial vein below the elbow level; either vein may

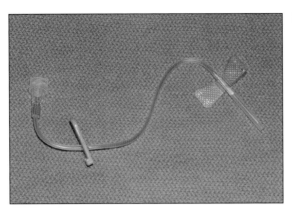

Fig A-5 Butterfly needle assembly.

be used. Veins at the back of the hand are very good for starting an intravenous access; however, the more peripheral nature of these veins and the thinness of the skin on the back of the hand cause them to collapse under the negative pressure of phlebotomy. They are therefore secondary choices for drawing blood for PRP preparation.

Phlebotomy Armamentaria

The armamentaria needed for drawing blood for PRP processing is a tourniquet, an alcohol or a betadine pad, and a phlebotomy needle/catheter. Two types of needle/catheter devices are in common use: the so-called butterfly needle (Fig A-5) and the catheter-over-needle (Fig A-6a). The butterfly needle was originally referred to as a *scalp vein needle* because it is easy to insert in infants, in whom scalp veins are the preferred phlebotomy site. This device consists of a beveled, stainless steel needle of an appropriate gauge, from which two plastic wings emerge at the shank. The hub of the needle is attached to a 6-inch length of tubing that can be connected to intravenous access tubing. The tubing attached to the hub of the needle will fill with blood once the needle is inserted into the lumen of the vein, confirming a successful venipuncture. The butterfly needle offers the operator excellent grasp and hence control via the wings. The wings also make it easy for the operator to securely tape the needle to the skin surface. The advantages of the butterfly system are that it is simple to learn, quick to perform, and an easy method for drawing blood. The disadvantage is that the sharp needle must remain within the vein, and any movement of the arm may result in perforation of the vein. This is especially likely if the vein crosses a joint, as occurs in the antecubital fossa. For this reason a catheter-over-needle device is preferred whenever intravenous access is needed for sedation procedures or the administration of medications.

As its name implies, the catheter-over-needle device is a stainless steel needle of an appropriate gauge over which a plastic catheter slides forward to enter the

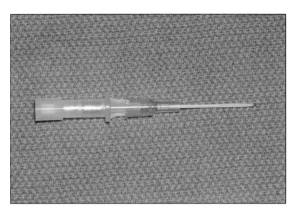

Fig A-6a A typical catheter-over-needle assembly.

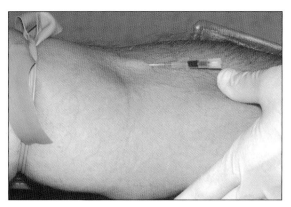

Fig A-6b The catheter-over-needle device shows blood filling the flashback chamber, indicating entry into the lumen of the vein.

Fig A-7 A 20-mL syringe is filled to 22 mL, of which 2 mL is the ACD-A and 20 mL is autologous blood. Note that the 60-mL preparation uses 7 mL of the ACD-A and 53 mL of autologous blood.

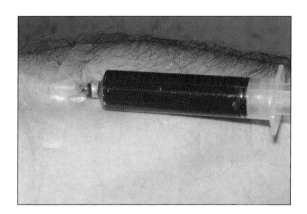

vein before the needle itself is withdrawn. (These devices are manufactured in sequences of even-numbered gauge sizes, whereas the butterfly devices are made in odd-numbered sequences.) This device has what is referred to as a *flashback chamber*, which fills with blood once the needle is inserted into the lumen of the vein (Fig A-6b). The back end of the catheter has a receptor port for connecting it to intravenous tubing. Because the needle-catheter combination must be positioned completely within the lumen of the vein and the vein stabilized for the catheter to advance over the needle, use of this device is slightly more difficult to learn; however, it is more suitable for the administration of intravenous sedation and medications as well as for long-term intravenous access.

Venipuncture procedure

If venipuncture is being performed for the purpose of processing PRP, the syringe that will be used for blood withdrawal must be prepared by aspirating 2 mL of anticoagulant citrate dextrose A (ACD-A) when drawing 20 mL of blood and 7 mL of ACD-A when drawing 60 mL of blood (Fig A-7).

Steps for Collecting Autologous Blood

1. **Assemble the armamentaria.** You will need gloves, syringes and/or blood-collecting tubes, needle device, tourniquet, 70% isopropyl alcohol pad or povidone-iodine pad, gauze, and tape (Fig A-8).

2. **Discuss the procedure with the patient and gain informed consent.** Tell the patient what you will be doing; why you are doing it; how much blood will be drawn; and what will be done with the blood after it is withdrawn. Allow the patient to ask questions. Assure the patient that you will use an aseptic technique. Obtain the patient's written consent. (A sample informed consent form is included at the end of this appendix.)

3. **Position the patient.** Seat the patient and choose the arm preferred by the patient or the one with the most prominent veins. Position the arm with the palm and the volar surface of the wrist up and with the arm in a straight line from shoulder to wrist. Make sure the arm is below the level of the heart so that the veins are full. Be sure that the light is coming in at an angle rather than straight over the vein to contrast the vein against the skin (Fig A-9).

4. **Select the vein site.** Apply the tourniquet and ask the patient to make a fist or squeeze a rubber ball, which will make the veins fill with blood and appear more prominent (Fig A-10). Choose a visible and palpable vein that is stable or that can be manually stabilized.

5. **Cleanse the venipuncture site with the alcohol pad or the povidone-iodine pad using circular motions.**

6. **Perform the venipuncture.** Tense the skin by pulling the skin back with your thumb. Insert the needle bevel up. Enter the skin at a shallow angle of 5 degrees to no more than 15 degrees (Fig A-11). Direct the needle to enter the vein from its top or side surface. You will feel a slight resistance as the needle goes through the dense skin tissue and the vein wall. A slight ease in this resistance indicates the presence of the needle in the lumen of the vein. If a butterfly device is used, tape the wings and the length of tubing before connecting the tubing to the syringe for blood withdrawal. If a catheter-over-needle device is used, advance the catheter to its hub and tape its smaller wings down with crossover taping before connecting the syringe for blood withdrawal (Fig A-12).

7. **Draw the blood.** For either system, allow a sufficient backflow of blood to force the air out of the needle hub and any tubing before connecting the syringe. Pull back the plunger slowly at an approximate rate of 1 mL/sec to prevent collapse of the vein or hemolysis of the red blood cells from an excessive amount of negative pressure. For the purposes of PRP processing, the blood will mix with the ACD-A as it is withdrawn (see Fig A-12). When the required amount of blood is obtained, release the tourniquet and disconnect the syringe. Then connect an intravenous solution line to the device and tape it down. If PRP processing is the sole purpose of the venipuncture, the needle/catheter device may be removed and a folded gauze applied to the site as a pressure bandage (Fig A-13). A simple bandage can also be used (Fig A-14). As soon as it is convenient, invert the syringe several times to mix the ADC-A and blood more completely.

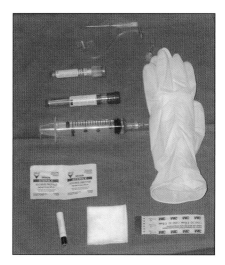

Fig A-8 Complete armamentaria for collecting autologous blood.

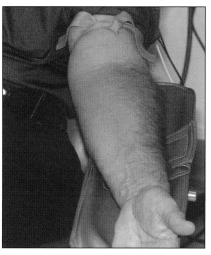

Fig A-9 The arm should be comfortably positioned with the palm facing upward, the elbow slightly bent in a straight line from shoulder to wrist and below the level of the heart.

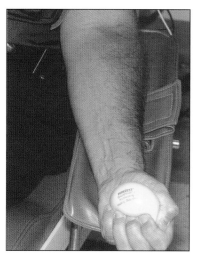

Fig A-10 Asking the patient to make a fist or squeeze a rubber ball will make the veins fill with blood and appear more prominent.

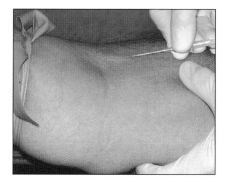

Fig A-11 The needle should enter the skin at a shallow angle (5 to 15 degrees).

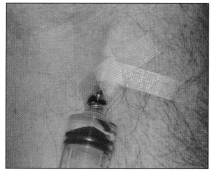

Fig A-12 The catheter-over-needle device is best secured with a crossover taping technique. When collecting autologous blood for PRP preparation, the ACD-A should already be in the syringe so that the blood will immediately mix with ACD-A and prevent coagulation.

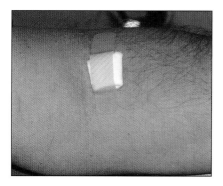

Fig A-13 A folded gauze beneath a plastic bandage serves as a simple, easy-to-use, and readily available pressure dressing following phlebotomy.

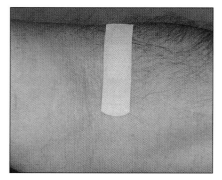

Fig A-14 A simple bandage alone also suffices for most phlebotomies.

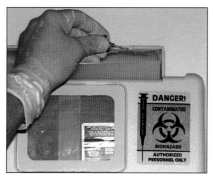

Fig A-15 Special sharps containers are available for disposing of phlebotomy needles. Use of such containers reduces the risk of inadvertent sticks from contaminated needles.

8. **Dispose of sharps and contaminated materials.** Place all needles in the devices designated for their disposal (Fig A-15). Place all remaining materials, such as gauze, sterilizing pads, syringes without needle, packaging, etc, in the red-colored containers designated for medical waste.

Potential Complications

True phlebotomy complications are extremely rare. Untold millions of venipunctures are accomplished every day with good patient acceptance and very few complications. The more likely complications of a single short-term venipuncture are pain and bruising (ecchymosis) at the venipuncture site. These are managed by time and/or heat and analgesics if necessary. If the pain persists and a palpable red and/or tender firmness develops at the venipuncture site, this would indicate a more serious complication, such as an infection. Such an infection could ascend proximally in the venous system and is known as a *septic thrombophlebitis*. This is initially managed with elevation of the site, heat, and staphylococcal antibiotic coverage as well as close follow-up. If the thrombophlebitis progresses or does not respond, in-patient management with blood culture studies and anticoagulation is required in addition to elevation, heat, and culture-directed antibiotics.

Another complication is nerve damage, which can affect the sensory or motor innervation of the hand or wrist. This is extremely unlikely if proper technique is followed because veins are more superficial than arteries, which are in turn much more superficial than nerves (see Fig A-2). In addition, a single-needle entry into a nerve without injection of a solution is not expected to be damaging to the nerve. Most post-venipuncture paresthesias are due to edema at the site rather than a nerve injury and will resolve within 2 to 3 weeks. If a paresthesia lasts longer than 3 weeks, an MRI study of the area and referral to an orthopedic hand specialist or a neurologist is recommended.

Still another remote potential complication is arterial puncture, which would be apparent by the spontaneous appearance or ready withdrawal of bright red blood under pressure. While arterial blood is suitable for PRP processing, the artery is not suitable for the administration of medications or solution. Therefore, the catheter should not be attached to intravenous tubing intended for such administration. If this is the purpose of the venipuncture, the needle should be withdrawn and direct digital pressure applied for 10 minutes followed by a folded gauze taped to the skin as a pressure dressing. The clinician should not be overly concerned about a short arterial puncture, which is intentionally carried out every day for arterial blood gas analysis, intensive care and anesthesia management, and invasive radiology procedures. Arteries recover just as readily as veins after a needle insertion; however, solutions or medications should never be administered arterially because they can compromise arterial flow to the arm and hand and ultimately result in tissue loss.

Consent Form for Phlebotomy and the Development of Platelet-Rich Plasma

I. Consent for Platelet-Rich Plasma

Dr _____ has recommended the use of platelet-rich plasma (PRP) to enhance your healing. PRP is a component of your own blood that contains growth factors known to stimulate bone and soft tissue healing. It is processed from your own blood in a sterile fashion and is therefore safe from transmission of diseases from others.

To process PRP, about 20 to 60 mL of blood (about ⅓ to ½ of a coffee cup) will be drawn from a vein using an aseptic technique. The risks associated with venipuncture are extremely small; however, there is a remote possibility that this invasive procedure may cause fainting, nausea, phlebitis, bruising, or nerve damage. Your blood will be processed for about 15 minutes in a device approved by the US Food and Drug Administration (FDA). It will then be activated and added to your surgical site to assist healing. To activate PRP, two drops of a calcium chloride solution are mixed with a clotting agent called thrombin, which is obtained from a commercial company that uses bovine (cow-derived) thrombin. When used to activate PRP, bovine thrombin is perfectly safe. However, your doctor can activate your PRP by alternative means at your request.

I, _____, voluntarily consent to the use of PRP as part of a wound-healing treatment plan. In order for my doctor to carry out this procedure, I consent to furnish 20 to 60 mL of my blood so that it can be processed in an FDA-approved device. After my blood is processed, a platelet concentrate will be produced. This material will be applied to my wound for the potential benefit of enhanced healing.

II. Explanation of Risks and Causes of Discomfort

I understand that PRP is applied topically and may cause some temporary local burning or irritation in some patients. I also understand that furnishing my blood will involve a needle stick into a vein in my arm or another location. While drawing blood involves minimal risk, there is a remote possibility that furnishing my blood may cause nausea, vomiting, fainting, dizziness, hematoma formation, bruising, blood loss, or infection. I may also experience discomfort from the needle stick at the puncture site.

III. Explanation of Benefits

I understand that PRP treatment is only part of my wound-healing program and that following all of the requirements of the treatment program is critical to the healing process. I also understand that the application of PRP has the potential to enhance and speed up my wound healing but is not a guarantee of healing.

IV. Additional Information

I am aware that I am free to withdraw my consent for treatment using this technology at any time. Withdrawal of my consent will not compromise my ability to continue to receive treatment. If I have questions during the course of my treatment, I can contact a staff member at _____ (telephone number).

V. Confidentiality

I authorize _____ to release my medical information to other healthcare providers to facilitate the coordination of my care. I understand that my medical information will be kept confidential to the extent required by law. Any information that does not identify me personally may be used for education, research, and publicity without any further permission.

VI. Understanding of This Form

I hereby acknowledge that I have been fully informed about the above-described procedure with its potential benefits and risks. I have had adequate time to reach my decision and have done so voluntarily. I am also aware that Dr _____ and/or the associates and staff of _____ will be available to answer any questions.

_____

Patient Signature   Date

_____

Witness Signature   Date

I have fully explained to _____ the nature and purpose of the above-described procedure and the risks involved in its performance. I have answered and will answer all questions to the best of my ability.

_____

Physician Signature   Date

Index

A

Access system, 44t, 46t-47t
ACD-A. *See* Anticoagulant citrate dextrose A.
Activation, 38, 38f, 41f
Adenosine diphosphate, 46
Allogeneic bone
  bone morphogenetic proteins in, 63
  description of, 27
  sinus lift grafting using, 63-65, 64f
Allogeneic dermis and coronally repositioned flaps for
    root coverage, 97, 98f-99f
Alopecia, 126, 128f
Alpha granules
  characteristics of, 4, 5f
  clotting process effects on, 5f
  growth factors secreted by, 9
Alveolar cleft grafting
  in bilateral cleft patients, 111, 115f
  bone grafting procedure for
    antibiotic prophylaxis, 111
    autogenous cancellous marrow used in, 111
    incisions, 111-112, 112f-114f
    platelet-rich plasma uses, 113f, 114
    recipient site preparation, 111
  complications of, 110
  goals of, 110
  indications for, 110
  lateral incisor removal, 110
  outcomes of, 114, 115f-116f
  patient age and, 110
  preoperative considerations, 110
  scar formation caused by, 110
Alveolar osteitis, 73-74, 75f
Alveolar ridge
  augmentation of. *See* Ridge augmentation.
  preservation of
    buccal wall blowout, 84, 85f
    complications that affect, 80
    graft materials, 82-83
    implant placement, 81-83, 83f-84f
    importance of, 80
    platelet-rich plasma for, 82-83
    teeth removal for, 80-81, 81f-82f
Antecubital veins, 33f
Anticoagulant citrate dextrose A
  calcium binding by, 38
  description of, 33, 33f, 35

mechanism of action, 38
  pH affected by, 74
  in phlebotomy procedure, 143-144
Arterial puncture, from phlebotomy, 146
Autogenous bone grafts
  biochemical environment of, 10f
  bone regenerated using, 62
  capillary penetration and profusion of, 11f
  guidelines for, 54t
  healing of, 10
  histomorphometry of, 17f
  macrophage's role in, 10, 12
  maturity index for, 16t
  optimization of, 62
  osteoid deposition, 12, 12f
  periodontal defects treated with, 78-79
  platelet-rich plasma–enhanced
    constructs, 40, 41f
    histomorphometry of, 17f
    maturity index for, 16t
    osteoprogenitor cells in, 15f, 27
    radiograph of, 16f
    trabecular bone values in, 15
  resorption-remodeling cycle, 12, 13f
  ridge augmentation using, 69
  sinus lift grafting use of, 54, 62, 63f
  trabecular bone value of, 55
Autogenous marrow grafts, 103
Autologous blood
  description of, 31
  phlebotomy collection procedure for, 143-144, 145f
Autologous platelet concentrate, 37

B

Bacteria, 3
Basilic vein, 141f
Blepharoplasty
  lower eyelid, 131-132, 132f
  side effects of, 130
  upper eyelid, 130-131, 131f
Blood, autologous
  description of, 31
  phlebotomy collection procedure for, 143-144, 145f
Blood clot
  cell ratios in, 9f
  in soft tissue healing, 18